Climate Change and Allergy

Editors

ROSALIND J. WRIGHT
JEFFREY G. DEMAIN

IMMUNOLOGY AND ALLERGY CLINICS OF NORTH AMERICA

www.immunology.theclinics.com

Consulting Editor
ROHIT KATIAL

February 2024 • Volume 44 • Number 1

ELSEVIER

1600 John F. Kennedy Boulevard • Suite 1800 • Philadelphia, Pennsylvania, 19103-2899

http://www.theclinics.com

IMMUNOLOGY AND ALLERGY CLINICS OF NORTH AMERICA Volume 44, Number 1

February 2024 ISSN 0889-8561, ISBN-13: 978-0-443-13011-3

Editor: Taylor Hayes
Developmental Editor: Nitesh Barthwal

Immunology and Allergy Clinics of North America (ISSN 0889–8561) is published quarterly by Elsevier Inc., 360 Park Avenue South, New York, NY 10010-1710. Months of issue are February, May, August, and November. Periodicals postage paid at New York, NY and additional mailing offices. Subscription prices are $375.00 per year for US individuals, $100.00 per year for US students and residents, $458.00 per year for Canadian individuals, $100.00 per year for Canadian students, $484.00 per year for international individuals, $220.00 per year for international students. For institutional access pricing please contact Customer Service via the contact information below. To receive student/resident rate, orders must be accompanied by name of affiliated institution, date of term, and the *signature* of program/residency coordinator on institution letterhead. Orders will be billed at individual rate until proof of status is received. Foreign air speed delivery is included in all *Clinics* subscription prices. All prices are subject to change without notice. **POSTMASTER**: Send address changes to *Immunology and Allergy Clinics of North America,* Elsevier Health Sciences Division, Subscription Customer Service, 3251 Riverport Lane, Maryland Heights, MO 63043. **Customer Service: 1-800-654-2452 (U.S. and Canada); 314-447-8871 (outside U.S. and Canada). Fax: 314-447-8029. E-mail:journalscustomerservice-usa@elsevier.com (for print support); journalsonlinesupport-usa@elsevier.com (for online support).**

Reprints. For copies of 100 or more, of articles in this publication, please contact the Commercial Reprints Department, Elsevier Inc., 360 Park Avenue South, New York, New York 10010-1710. Tel. 212-633-3874, Fax: 212-633-3820, E-mail: reprints@elsevier.com.

Immunology and Allergy Clinics of North America is covered in MEDLINE/PubMed (Index Medicus), Current Contents/Life Sciences, Science Citation Index, ISI/BIOMED, Chemical Abstracts, and EMBASE/Excerpta Medica.

Contributors

CONSULTING EDITOR

ROHIT KATIAL, MD, FAAAAI, FACAAI, FACP
Professor of Medicine, Associate Vice President of Education, Director, Center for Clinical Immunology, Irene J. & Dr. Abraham E. Goldminz, Chair in Immunology and Respiratory Medicine, Division of Allergy and Clinical Immunology, Department of Medicine, National Jewish Health, University of Colorado, Denver, Colorado, USA

EDITORS

ROSALIND J. WRIGHT, MD, MPH
Professor, Department of Environmental Medicine and Public Health, Institute for Exposomic Research, Icahn School of Medicine at Mount Sinai, New York, New York, USA

JEFFREY G. DEMAIN, MD
Clinical Professor, Department of Pediatrics, University of Washington, Seattle, Washington, USA; WWAMI School of Medicine, University of Alaska, Anchorage, Alaska, USA

AUTHORS

HERESH AMINI, PhD
Associate Professor, Department of Environmental Medicine and Public Health, Institute for Exposomic Research, Icahn School of Medicine at Mount Sinai, New York, New York, USA

MOHAMAD AMINI, MD
Dermatologist, Department of Dermatology, Besat Hospital, Kurdistan University of Medical Sciences, Sanandaj, Iran

JONATHAN A. BERNSTEIN, MD
Professor of Medicine, Division of Rheumatology, Allergy and Immunology, Department of Internal Medicine, University of Cincinnati College of Medicine, Cincinnati, Ohio, USA

YOUNG-JIN CHOI, MD, PhD
Assistant Professor, Department of Pediatrics, College of Medicine, Hanyang University, Seoul, Korea; Department of Pediatrics, Hanyang University Guri Hospital, Guri, Gyunggi-Do, Korea

KECIA N. CARROLL, MD, MPH
Professor, Division of General Pediatrics, Departments of Pediatrics and Environmental Medicine and Public Health, Icahn School of Medicine at Mount Sinai, New York, New York, USA

ALINA GHERASIM, MD
Clinical Research Physician, ALYATEC Environmental Exposure Chamber, Strasbourg, France

ITAI KLOOG, PhD
Professor, Department of Environmental Medicine and Public Health, Institute for Exposomic Research, Icahn School of Medicine at Mount Sinai, New York, New York, USA; Department of Geography and Environmental Development, Ben-Gurion University, Beer Sheva, Israel

ALISON G. LEE, MD, MS
Associate Professor, Division of Pulmonary, Critical Care and Sleep Medicine, Icahn School of Medicine at Mount Sinai, New York, New York, USA

ASHLEY SANG EUN LEE, MD
Clinical Fellow, Division of Allergy and Immunology, Icahn School of Medicine at Mount Sinai; Department of Pediatrics, Jaffe Food Allergy Institute, New York, New York, USA

JENNILEE LUEDDERS, MD
Fellow, Division of Allergy and Immunology, Department of Internal Medicine, University of Nebraska Medical Center, Omaha, Nebraska, USA

PABLO E. MOREJÓN-JARAMILLO, MD
Post-Doctoral Research Fellow, Division of Pulmonary and Critical Care Medicine, Department of Medicine, Beth Israel Deaconess Medical Center, Boston, Massachusetts, USA

NICHOLAS J. NASSIKAS, MD
Instructor in Medicine, Division of Pulmonary and Critical Care Medicine, Department of Medicine, Harvard Medical School, Beth Israel Deaconess Medical Center, Boston, Massachusetts, USA

JAE-WON OH, MD, PhD, FAAAAI
Professor, Head of Department (Pediatrics), Department of Pediatrics, College of Medicine, Hanyang University, Seoul, Korea; Department of Pediatrics, Hanyang University Guri Hospital, Guri, Gyunggi-Do, Korea

DAVID B. PEDEN, MD, MS
Senior Associate Dean for Translational Research, UNC School of Medicinemedical Director, Division of Pediatric Allergy and Immunology, Center for Environmental Medicine, Asthma and Lung Biology, The University of North Carolina at Chapel Hill, UNC School of Medicine, Chapel Hill, North Carolina, USA

JILL A. POOLE, MD
Professor, Division of Allergy and Immunology, Department of Internal Medicine, University of Nebraska Medical Center, Omaha, Nebraska, USA

NICOLE RAMSEY, MD, PhD
Assistant Professor, Division of Allergy and Immunology, Department of Pediatrics, Icahn School of Medicine at Mount Sinai, Jaffe Food Allergy Institute, New York, New York, USA

MARY B. RICE, MD, MPH
Associate Professor of Medicine, Division of Pulmonary and Critical Care Medicine, Department of Medicine, Harvard Medical School, Beth Israel Deaconess Medical Center, Boston, Massachusetts, USA

ANDREW C. RORIE, MD
Assistant Professor, Division of Allergy and Immunology, Department of Internal Medicine, University of Nebraska Medical Center, Omaha, Nebraska, USA

ROBERT O. WRIGHT, MD, MPH
Professor and Pediatrician, Department of Environmental Medicine and Public Health, Institute for Exposomic Research, Icahn School of Medicine at Mount Sinai, New York, New York, USA

XUEYING ZHANG, PhD
Instructor, Department of Environmental Medicine and Public Health, Institute for Exposomic Research, Icahn School of Medicine at Mount Sinai, New York, New York, USA

Contents

> Climate change is a major threat to human respiratory health and associated allergic disorders given its broad impact on the exposome. Climate change can affect exposure to allergens, such as pollen, dust mites, molds, as well as other factors such as temperature, air pollution, and nutritional factors, which synergistically impact the immune response to these allergens. Exposome change can differentially exacerbate allergic reactions across subgroups of populations, especially those who are more vulnerable to environmental stressors. Understanding links between climate change and health impacts can help inform how to protect individuals and vulnerable populations from adverse health effects.

> Air pollution is a risk factor for asthma and respiratory infection. Avoidance of air pollution is the best approach to mitigating the impacts of pollution. Personal preventive strategies are possible, but policy interventions are the most effective ways to prevent pollution and its effect on asthma and respiratory infection.

> The objective of this article is to review recent literature on the implications of extreme weather events such as thunderstorms, wildfires, tropical cyclones, freshwater flooding, and temperature extremes in relationship to asthma symptoms. Several studies have shown worsening of asthma symptoms with thunderstorms, wildfires, tropical cyclones, freshwater flooding, and temperature extremes. In particular, thunderstorm asthma can be exacerbated by certain factors such as temperature, precipitation, and allergen sensitization. Therefore, it is imperative that the allergy and immunology community be aware of the health effects associated with these extreme weather events in order to educate patients and engage in mitigation strategies.

> The U.S. Global Change Research Program, Fourth National Climate Assessment reports that it is extremely likely that human activities, especially

temperature. The rise in global temperature has led to an increase in heat waves and extreme weather events, which pose serious risks to respiratory health. Accurately assessing the effects of air temperature on respiratory health requires a comprehensive approach that incorporates fine-scale exposure assessment to characterize the geospatial environment impacting population health. Recent advances in open-source earth observation data have allowed for improved exposure assessment through temperature modeling.

Clinical Medicine and Climate Change

Pablo E. Morejón-Jaramillo, Nicholas J. Nassikas, and Mary B. Rice

The health care system contributes substantially to global greenhouse gas emissions, a driver of climate change. At the same time, climate change has caused disruptions in health care delivery. In this article, the authors describe both how the health care industry contributes to climate change and how climate change affects patient care. The authors also provide clinical recommendations for health care practitioners to counsel patients on health effects of climate change and underscore the need for developing the workforce to respond to unique health care delivery challenges resulting from climate-related factors.

IMMUNOLOGY AND ALLERGY CLINICS OF NORTH AMERICA

SERIES OF RELATED INTEREST

Medical Clinics
https://www.medical.theclinics.com/

THE CLINICS ARE AVAILABLE ONLINE!
Access your subscription at:
www.theclinics.com

Preface

Growing Impact of Climate Change on Respiratory Health and Related Allergic Disorders: Need for Health Systems to Prepare

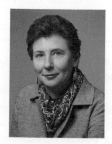
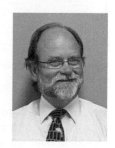

Rosalind J. Wright, MD, MPH   Jeffrey G. Demain, MD

Editors

The World Health Organization has identified climate change as the biggest health threat facing humanity.[1] The days of a polar bear stranded on an ice flow as the icon of global warming have passed. What scientists have predicted for decades has now become a reality. We are now witnessing the growing impact on human health as a result of our changing climate, our warming planet, and continued increase in greenhouse gas emissions.

Asthma and related respiratory disorders have also increased in recent decades coinciding with climate related changes in our ecosystem. Our understanding of the environmental influences on both the onset of new disease and the exacerbation of established respiratory and related allergic disorders is growing increasingly complex with an expanding list of recognized environmental, microbial, social, and nutritional exposures playing a role (eg, ambient and indoor pollutants and aeroallergens, viral infections, molds, psychological stress, diet quality, chemical toxins such as trace metals). Programming effects result from toxin-induced shifts in a host of molecular, cellular, and physiologic states and their interacting systems.[2] If exposures occur in critical windows of development when these systems are most vulnerable to alteration, especially during fetal development in utero or early childhood, there can be lifelong impacts on respiratory health and related allergic diseases, magnifying their impact.[3]

We begin this collection with an overview of the complex ways climate change effects on our social and physical environment, both directly and indirectly, impact respiratory health and related allergic disorders. As depicted in **Fig. 1**, broad ranging

Immunol Allergy Clin N Am 44 (2024) xi–xv
https://doi.org/10.1016/j.iac.2023.10.001
0889-8561/24/© 2023 Published by Elsevier Inc.

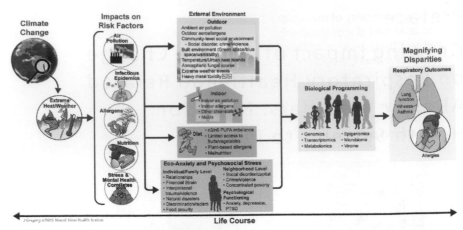

Fig. 1. Climate change, environmental impacts, and cumulative risk for respiratory outcomes.

effects of climate change consequent to rising global average temperatures, increasing carbon dioxide (CO_2) in the atmosphere, consequent weather changes (ie, extreme weather events including heat waves, droughts or floods, hurricanes), and disrupted ecosystem functioning and biodiversity have alarming potential for magnifying respiratory and related allergic disease burden worldwide.[4] Attention has focused on the influence of climate change on changing exposure to chemical pollutants and aeroallergens in both ambient air and the indoor environment.[5,6] For example, rising air temperatures and CO_2 concentrations contribute to increased pollen production and prolonged duration of pollen seasons, resulting in higher prevalence and greater severity of allergic and other respiratory disorders. Alarmingly, current models predict that ragweed levels will increase by more than four times over the next 30 years. More recent focus brings attention to links between rising CO_2 due to fossil fuel burning and indoor pollution. Extreme weather events, including thunderstorms and tropical storm systems, can lead to proliferation of microbial and mold growth in homes impacted by flooding. In another global trend, unwanted trace metals and persistent organic pollutants are increasingly detected in vegetables and drinking water[7] due to changing climate conditions, including those toxins previously associated with respiratory disease morbidity. For example, with climate-associated drying up of water bodies and reservoirs, sediments become soils, which can be redistributed by winds and other storm-related factors, enhancing soil-bound heavy metals contamination of our environment, including the air we breathe. While these factors are important drivers of the increased burden of respiratory disease, additional climate change phenomena further contribute to impacts on respiratory health.

Climate change is anticipated to continue to alter availability to as well as nutritional value of a range of food sources[8,9] that can impact asthma and related allergic diseases.[10] The loss of biodiversity related to climate change may affect the microbiome, contributing to inflammatory respiratory disorders. Immunologic disorders, such as plant food allergies linked to greater asthma risk, are also impacted. For example, studies have found that increases in CO_2 and temperature are correlated with changes in the composition of the peanut, making it more immunogenic. Long-chain polyunsaturated fatty acid (PUFA) intake has been of great interest to the allergy community given their influence on oxidative stress and immune deviation that contribute to asthma programming, lung development, and skin or aeroallergies.

The global availability of marine and plant oils, major dietary sources of eicosapen-taenoic acid and docosahexaenoic acid, which have anti-inflammatory properties as well as others promoting inflammation, is impacted by climate factors.[11] Intake of a range of micronutrients plays a role in both disease onset and expression of disease over the life span.[12] As discussed in more detail by Carroll in this collection, research demonstrates protective effects of omega-3 (n-3) PUFA intake on wheeze or asthma. Over time, dietary patterns have changed, with an increase in proinflam-matory omega-6 PUFA intake relative to anti-inflammatory n-3 PUFAs. Moreover, these changing patterns in PUFA intake have paralleled increases in asthma preva-lence. Climate warming and consequent increasing water temperatures are pro-jected to alter the biochemical composition of phytoplankton, a main source of n-3 long-chain essential fatty acids in aquatic ecosystems, with cascading effects that will further exacerbate this imbalance in human micronutrient intakes that impact health.[13]

Populations experiencing extreme weather events and extreme heat due to climate warming are also more vulnerable to developing mental health disorders (anxiety, depression) that impact chronic respiratory disorders across the life course. Effects on psychological well-being can be direct (heat stress, exposure to traumatic events, including natural disasters) and indirect (economic loss, threats to health and well-being, displacement or forced migration, collective violence). Research increas-ingly links climate-related phenomena with being more likely to experience stress and social consequences, including increased collective and interpersonal violence exposure.[14–16] Psychological functioning and increased exposure to chronic stressors, including violence, have been linked to respiratory disease expression, including intergenerational effects.[3] These impacts will also disproportionately affect those already most vulnerable living in less-resourced communities and regions of the world.

In addition, individuals are not exposed to a single factor or chemical at a given time, but to complex mixtures that interact with compound risk. For example, air pollution from fossil fuel burning and traffic-related emissions can alter respiratory defense mechanisms and act synergistically with allergens to enhance immunoge-nicity to worsen outcomes.[17] Although traditional disciplinary research theory and methods have focused separately on how social and physical environmental factors affect asthma and related allergic disorders, evolving research underscores impor-tant integrated effects. Social phenomena and related nonchemical stressors covary and interact with chemical and physical stressors to influence disease expression.[18] Also, anticipated climate impacts will disproportionately affect regions and popula-tions where the prevalence of both toxic exposures discussed herein and disease burden is already high and/or increasing.[19,20] This will amplify already unacceptable and costly health disparities. We must consider a more comprehensive framework of environmental influences on respiratory health, as depicted in **Fig. 1** and dis-cussed in greater depth in the collection of articles herein, in order to more fully comprehend the impact of climate change on disease expression over the life course.

Finally, we end this collection with a section providing clinical recommenda-tions for health care practitioners to counsel patients on health effects of climate change and underscore the need for developing the workforce needed to respond to unique health care delivery challenges resulting from climate-related factors. This section also acknowledges how health care systems can change op-erations to minimize their own contribution to climate crises and the impacts on health.

ACKNOWLEDGEMENT

During preparation of this manuscript RJ Wright was supported through the National Institutes of Health, Bethesda, MD, USA by the National Center for Advancing Translational Sciences (NCATS) Clinical and Translational Science Award (CTSA) Program grant UL1TR004419.

Rosalind J. Wright, MD, MPH
Department of Environmental Medicine
and Public Health
Institute for Exposomic Research
Icahn School of Medicine at
Mount Sinai
One Gustave L. Levy Place
New York, NY, 10029, USA

Jeffrey G. Demain, MD
Department of Pediatrics
University of Washington
Seattle WA, USA

WWAMI School of Medicine
University of Alaska
Anchorage, AK 99516, USA

E-mail addresses:
rosalind.wright@mssm.edu (R.J. Wright)
jeff@demain.pro (J.G. Demain)

REFERENCES

1. Addressing climate change. Supplement to the WHO water, sanitation and hygiene strategy 2018–2025. Geneva: World Health Organization; 2023.
2. Murrison LB, Brandt EB, Myers JB, et al. Environmental exposures and mechanisms in allergy and asthma development. J Clin Invest 2019;129:1504–15. PMC6436881.
3. Rosa MJ, Lee AG, Wright RJ. Evidence establishing a link between prenatal and early-life stress and asthma development. Curr Opin Allergy Clin Immunol 2018; 18:148–58. PMC5835351.
4. Patz JA, Frumkin H, Holloway T, et al. Climate change: challenges and opportunities for global health. JAMA 2014;312(15):1565–80.
5. D'Amato G, Chong-Neto HJ, Monge Ortega OP, et al. The effects of climate change on respiratory allergy and asthma induced by pollen and mold allergens. Allergy 2020.
6. Poole JA, Barnes CS, Demain JG, et al. Impact of weather and climate change with indoor and outdoor air quality in asthma: a work group report of the AAAAI Environmental Exposure and Respiratory Health Committee. J Allergy Clin Immunol 2019;143:1702–10.
7. Ondrasek G, Bakic Begic H, Zovko M, et al. Biogeochemistry of soil organic matter in agroecosystems & environmental implications. Sci Total Environ 2019;658: 1559–73.
8. Nawaz M, Sun J, Shabbir S, et al. A review of plants strategies to resist biotic and abiotic environmental stressors. Sci Total Environ 2023;900:165832.

9. Williams CE, Williams CL, Logan ML. Climate change is not just global warming: multidimensional impacts on animal gut microbiota. Microb Biotechnol 2023;16: 1736–44. PMC10443335.
10. Haahtela T. A biodiversity hypothesis. Allergy 2019;74:1445–56.
11. Tan K, Ransangan J, Tan K, et al. The impact of climate change on Omega-3 long-chain polyunsaturated fatty acids in bivalves. Crit Rev Food Sci Nutr 2023;1–11.
12. Barros R, Moreira A, Padrao P, et al. Dietary patterns and asthma prevalence, incidence and control. Clin Exp Allergy 2015;45:1673–80.
13. Hixson SM, Arts MT. Climate warming is predicted to reduce omega-3, long-chain, polyunsaturated fatty acid production in phytoplankton. Glob Chang Biol 2016;22:2744–55.
14. Mares D. Climate change and levels of violence in socially disadvantaged neighborhood groups. J Urban Health 2013;90:768–83. PMC3732690.
15. Xu R, Xiong X, Abramson MJ, et al. Ambient temperature and intentional homicide: a multi-city case-crossover study in the US. Environ Int 2020;143:105992.
16. Levy BS, Sidel VW, Patz JA. Climate change and collective violence. Annu Rev Public Health 2017;38:241–57. PMC6098709.
17. Naclerio R, Ansotegui IJ, Bousquet J, et al. International expert consensus on the management of allergic rhinitis (AR) aggravated by air pollutants: impact of air pollution on patients with AR: current knowledge and future strategies. World Allergy Organ J 2020;13:100106. PMC7132263.
18. Wright RJ. Moving towards making social toxins mainstream in children's environmental health. Curr Opin Pediatr 2009;21:222–9. PMC2752500.
19. Levy BS, Patz JA. Climate change, human rights, and social justice. Ann Glob Health 2015;81:310–22.
20. Thomas K, Hardy RD, Lazrus H, et al. Explaining differential vulnerability to climate change: a social science review. Wiley Interdiscip Rev Clim Change 2019;10:e565. PMC6472565.

Climate Change, Exposome Change, and Allergy
A Review

Heresh Amini, PhD[a],*, Mohamad Amini, MD[b], Robert O. Wright, MD, MPH[a]

KEYWORDS

- Climate change • Exposome change • Allergy • Dermatitis • Rhinitis

KEY POINTS

- Climate change impacts a host of environmental influences on respiratory health and related allergic disorders.
- Vulnerable populations (the elderly, children, or pregnant women), especially of low socioeconomic status, will be disproportionately impacted by climate-related environmental shifts.
- Our understanding of the broad impact of climate change on disease risk will be advanced through emerging technologies and data science advancements using an exposome framework.

BACKGROUND

Climate change (CC) involves changes in various aspects of the climate system, such as temperature, precipitation, wind patterns, ocean currents, and atmospheric composition.[1] While CC has natural causes, such as changes in solar activity or volcanic eruptions, the leading cause is human activities, especially the burning of fossil fuels like coal, oil, and gas. These activities emit greenhouse gases, such as carbon dioxide (CO_2) and methane, into the atmosphere, which act like a blanket and trap heat on the planet. Greenhouse gas concentrations are currently at their highest levels and emissions continue to rise. Consequently, the Earth is now about 1.1°C warmer than it was in the late 1800s.[2] The last decade (2011–2020) was the warmest on record, and surface temperature records are moving year after year.[3] The impacts of CC are already visible and widespread, such as melting ice caps and glaciers, more

[a] Department of Environmental Medicine and Public Health, Institute for Exposomic Research, Icahn School of Medicine at Mount Sinai, 1 Gustave L. Levy Pl, New York, NY 10029, USA; [b] Department of Dermatology, Besat Hospital, Kurdistan University of Medical Sciences, Sanandaj, Iran
* Corresponding author.
E-mail address: heresh.amini@mssm.edu

Immunol Allergy Clin N Am 44 (2024) 1–13
https://doi.org/10.1016/j.iac.2023.09.003
0889-8561/24/© 2023 Elsevier Inc. All rights reserved.

frequent and intense extreme weather events, droughts, floods, and wildfires. CC also poses serious challenges for food security, water availability, energy supply, migration patterns, human security, and economic development. Some regions and populations are more vulnerable to climate impacts than others.

Allergies affect millions of people around the world and consist of a maladaptive immune system reaction to foreign substances or allergens, such as pollen, food, or insect venom. Allergens cause various symptoms depending on the type and severity of the allergic disorder including sneezing, itching, swelling, rash, and, in severe cases, difficulty breathing.

A multitude of social, chemical, nutritional, and microbial environmental exposures influence allergic and nonallergic respiratory disease programming and natural history. Clinical manifestations result from toxin-induced shifts in a host of molecular, cellular, and physiologic states and their interacting systems. Moreover, individuals are not exposed to a single environmental factor at a given time but to complex mixtures. This complexity has fostered the concept of the *exposome*, a framework that considers multiple external exposures as well as the internal environment indexed via physiologic response biomarkers, accounting for exposure timing.[4] Exposome is proposed as a complement to the human genome, recognizing that genetic factors alone cannot explain the causes of the majority of chronic diseases.[5] A systematic approach to measuring environmental exposures could fill this knowledge gap and identify potential prevention strategies. The exposome includes external factors, such as air pollution, temperature, humidity, chemicals, radiation, or socioeconomic status (SES), and internal factors and biological responses, such as metabolism, hormones, oxidative stress, inflammation, and gut microbiota.[6] While acceptance was slow at first, in recent years exposomics has received a large amount of attention from the scientific community.

This article aims to provide a review of how CC affects exposome change (EC) and how this influences the prevalence and severity of various allergic conditions.

AN OVERVIEW OF ALLERGY AND ITS TYPES

Allergic reactions can be classified into 4 types based on the mechanism of the immune response: type I (anaphylactic), type II (cytotoxic), type III (immunocomplex), and type IV (cell-mediated).[7] Types I, II, and III are immediate reactions that occur within 24 hours of exposure to the allergen. Type IV is a delayed reaction that usually appears after 24 hours of exposure.[7] The most common types of allergies are indoor/outdoor allergies (such as hay fever/allergic rhinitis or nasal allergies), skin allergies (such as eczema, hives, or contact dermatitis), food allergies, or insect allergies (such as bee stings or fire ant bites). Seasonal allergies are caused by airborne particles, such as pollen, that trigger symptoms like sneezing, runny nose, and itchy eyes and vary by calendar months reflecting when different types of pollen are released.[8] Mold allergies arise from fungi that grow in damp places, such as bathrooms, basements, or outdoors.[9] Insect allergies are caused by being stung or bitten by insects that inject venom or saliva eliciting swelling, itching, hives, and even anaphylaxis with the most common insects being bees, wasps, fire ants, or mosquitoes.[10]

BURDEN OF DISEASE DUE TO ALLERGY

Allergy and related respiratory disorders such as asthma result in significant morbidity, mortality, and economic burden. Allergic diseases vary depending on the type of allergy, the geographic region, the age group, and the method of diagnosis, with multiple allergies often coexisting in the same individual, increasing the complexity and severity of the condition. Allergies are often comorbid with asthma, chronic rhinitis, and atopic dermatitis (AD).[11] Allergies are the greatest contributor to the disability-adjusted life years (DALYs) of skin diseases.[12] The regional burden of disease due to allergies varies depending on the type and severity of allergic diseases, as well as the availability and accessibility of health care services. The World Bank regions with the highest age-standardized DALYs for both sexes due to AD in 2019 are shown in **Fig. 1**. In the United States, about 26% of adults and 20% of children have been diagnosed with allergic conditions, with similar rates in Europe.[13] The cost of allergic diseases is in the billions and includes medical care as well as lost productivity and reduced quality of life.[14] Allergic diseases can also impair the physical, psychological, and social well-being of affected individuals and their families.[15] Reduced sleep quality and daytime functioning due to nasal congestion, coughing, or itching; increased anxiety and depression due to fear of exposure to allergens or anaphylaxis; and increased school absenteeism and lower academic performance due to asthma or allergic rhinitis are just some examples.[16]

CLIMATE CHANGE, EXPOSOME CHANGE, AND ALLERGY
Impacts on Temperature, Humidity, Air Pollution, Pollen, and Allergy

Human activities have caused the global average annual temperature to rise by nearly 2° F (1.1° C) since preindustrial times.[17] These impacts are uneven with many regions warming faster than others. It is noteworthy that CC is not evenly distributed globally and may actually cause colder, extended winter seasons in some parts of the world. This adds complexity to CC research as low and high ambient temperatures have been both associated with increased cardiorespiratory hospitalization in previous studies.[18,19]

With CC, atmospheric pressure and circulation patterns change, leading to more frequent extreme weather events. Melting ice sheets, rising sea levels, more frequent and intense heat waves, droughts, wildfires, storms, and floods are becoming more commonplace. These events can have serious consequences for human and natural systems.

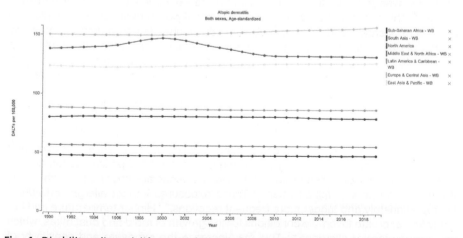

Fig. 1. Disability-adjusted life years (DALYs) for atopic dermatitis for both sexes, age-standardized across World Bank (WB) regions. (Source: Institute for Health Metrics Evaluation. Used with permission. All rights reserved.)

CC is not only affecting global temperature but also the amount of water vapor in the air. This has significant impacts on both the frequency and intensity of extreme weather events, such as heavy rainfall and heatwaves. According to Williams and colleagues, specific humidity has increased over both land and ocean as the air has warmed. However, relative humidity has decreased over land as it has warmed faster than the ocean.[20] This means that the air over land is relatively drier over time even though the capacity to hold water vapor has increased. This creates a humidity paradox that affects the Earth's water cycle and the energy balance explaining why some geographic areas have higher rainfall while others experience drought. Higher specific humidity can lead to heavier rainfall events and more flooding, as more water vapor is available to condense and precipitate. Higher specific humidity combined with higher temperatures can cause heat stress, a condition that reduces the ability of the body to cool down by sweating and can be fatal in some cases.[21]

While air pollution is a major cause of CC, the effects are bidirectional with CC also increasing air pollution levels across the world. This is because CC alters weather patterns that affect the dispersion of pollutants in the atmosphere. Moreover, CC can increase the frequency and intensity of wildfires, dust storms, and other events that produce large amounts of smoke and particulate matter (PM).[22] Short and long-term exposure to air pollution has been associated with higher mortality and morbidity consistently across the world.[23-27] Higher temperatures increase the formation of ground-level ozone, which can cause respiratory problems and damage crops.[28] Previous researchers have investigated what is known as the "climate penalty" for air pollution, defined as the additional increases in air pollution relative to trends assuming constant weather conditions.[29] This climate penalty in the United States has led to increases in ozone associated with an additional 290 (95% confidence interval [CI]: 80, 510) premature mortalities annually.[29] For fine PM ≤ 2.5 μm ($PM_{2.5}$) it was linked to 770 (95% CI: 190, 1350) excess annual deaths.[29] Numerous studies have also documented substantial impacts of wildfire smoke, which is expected to increase due to CC,[30] on a spectrum of health outcomes, such as exacerbations of asthma, chronic obstructive pulmonary disease, and respiratory infections.[25,31,32]

CC, rising CO_2 concentrations, and increased temperature have significant impacts on pollen production and distribution.[33,34] Higher temperatures cause plants, trees, grass, and weeds to produce more pollen and release it earlier than their particular season.[35] This extends the duration and intensity of pollen exposure for people who suffer from allergies and asthma.[36] Additionally, higher temperatures increase the amount of ozone and other pollutants in the air, which worsen the effects of pollen on respiratory health.[37] CC also affects the geographic range and the diversity of pollen sources, potentially exposing people to new allergens that they are not accustomed to.[38]

The impact of CC on the external exposome and its impact on allergy are complex and affect geographic locations and vulnerable populations differently.[39] Altered outdoor and indoor exposomes, such as temperature, humidity, air pollution, and so forth, affect allergies (eg, respiratory or skin allergies) in many ways. As explained earlier, higher temperatures along with rising CO_2 extend the pollen season and increase the amount of pollen produced by plants, especially ragweed, which is one of the main triggers of fall allergies.[38] These exposures impact allergic individuals disproportionately and trigger more frequent reactions.[40] Higher temperature and humidity further create favorable conditions for the growth of mold and dust mites, which are common indoor allergens.[41] This may increase the exposure and sensitivity of allergic individuals to these allergens and trigger allergic reactions.[9,42] Another potential effect of CC is triggering or exacerbation of temperature-based urticaria, a type of allergic reaction that occurs when the skin is exposed to cold or hot temperatures in sensitive individuals. Cold or hot urticaria cause itching, swelling, redness and hives on the skin, and, while rare, in severe cases, anaphylaxis.[43] Higher temperatures can increase the production of proinflammatory cytokines and reactive oxygen species, which damage cells and tissues.[44]

Higher temperatures, as discussed in the previous sections, may further increase the levels of some air pollutants, such as ozone and PM, which irritate the respiratory system, breaking down defensive barriers and making individuals more sensitive to allergens and allergic symptoms.[45] Air pollution is an important risk factor for AD.[46] Possible mechanisms for this association include increased water loss, physicochemical injury, effects on skin microflora, and damage to the skin barrier through oxidative stress. Importantly, immune dysregulation can be triggered by oxidative stress, causing increased sensitization to allergens.[46] Short-term exposure to air pollution has been associated with psoriasis flare.[47] Long-term exposure to air pollution has also been associated with increased prevalence of psoriasis and eczema in the United States, with a magnitude comparable to the risk associated with smoking.[48] Increased air pollution and pollen under CC and complex interactions with other allergens could trigger inflammatory responses and oxidative stress leading to aggravated allergies and higher burden of allergic disease worldwide.[49]

Prior research has shown that air pollution can impair vitamin D production directly by blocking ultraviolet B photons (eg, under smoke or dust pollution) or indirectly by decreasing outdoor activity and less exposure to ambient ultraviolet radiation.[50] AD, asthma, and respiratory infection have been associated with vitamin D deficiency across several studies.[51]

Impacts on Electromagnetic Field Radiation

Electromagnetic field (EMF) radiation arises from electrical devices and power lines and can affect living organisms. Under the changing climate, the demand for electricity and the use of electrical devices, especially for cooling and heating purposes, will increase and may increase population-level EMF exposure. CC may also alter natural background EMF levels via changes in atmospheric and geomagnetic conditions, such as solar storms and lightning activity. The EMF exposure can cause changes in cell function, gene expression, hormone levels, and disturbance of the immune system.[52] Most interestingly, EMF radiation may also trigger a condition called electromagnetic hypersensitivity or electrohypersensitivity (EHS), which is a perceived sensitivity to EMFs emitted by various sources such as power lines, cell phones, computers, and microwaves.[53] Symptoms of EHS include nausea, vomiting, diarrhea, headache, fever, dizziness, disorientation, weakness, fatigue, hair loss, and bloody vomit and stools from internal bleeding.[54] Anyhow, whether EHS is caused by EMFs or that it is a true allergic reaction is still an area of investigation.

Impacts on Chemical Exposure

CC may indirectly increase exposure to chemicals that could harm our bodies and ecosystems. For example, floods may cause chemicals stored in landfills, tanks, or debris to leak or spread to new areas.[55] The melting of permafrost in Alaska may release chemicals that were previously frozen and volatile chemicals such as mercury will be carried to different geographic areas based on temperature.[56] CC is able to impact internal hormones by altering the natural or human-made chemicals that interact with the endocrine system, called endocrine-disrupting chemicals (EDCs).[57] EDCs have been found in many products, such as plastics, pesticides, cosmetics, and pharmaceuticals, and can contaminate water, air, and soil.[58] Some examples of

EDCs are atrazine, bisphenol A (BPA), and phthalates.[59] The EDCs mimic, block, or interfere with the body's hormones and cause various health problems.[60] As an example, CC can increase the population exposure to the herbicide atrazine where higher temperatures increase the volatility and evaporation of atrazine from soil and water surfaces, leading to greater atmospheric deposition. Increased rainfall and flooding also can increase the runoff of atrazine from agricultural fields into surface water and groundwater.[61] These scenarios can result in higher levels of atrazine in humans. Atrazine can affect the immune system by altering the production of cytokines, chemokines, and immunoglobulins and modulating the function of macrophages, T cells, and B cells, affecting a range of allergies.[62]

As another example, CC can make people more exposed to BPA. Higher temperatures can make BPA leach out of plastic products into food or water, and more rain and flooding can make BPA wash away from landfills into surface water. These situations again can lead to higher levels of BPA in humans. BPA may trigger systemic para-inflammation in epithelial tissues, such as the skin, gut, and lungs.[63] Para-inflammation is a low-grade chronic inflammatory state that is normally protective against stress or injury but can become maladaptive if prolonged or excessive.[64] Para-inflammation can impair the epithelial barrier function and increase the permeability to allergens and pathogens.[65] It can also activate innate immune cells and induce the production of proinflammatory cytokines, such as interleukin 6 and tumor necrosis factor-α, which can promote allergic inflammation.[66]

Plastics are ubiquitous, and exacerbated degradation of discarded plastics yields nanoplastic particles that are incorporated into microorganisms under different temperature levels in a dose-dependent manner.[67] Emission of micro/nanoplastics along with different chemicals during wildfires and burning of plastic material is an underappreciated impact of CC as they can induce an immune response leading to cellular toxicity and genotoxicity.[68] CC-induced increased temperature may result in increased release of chemicals from plastics, increasing the risk of exposure.[69] Some of these chemicals, such as phthalates, interfere with the endocrine system and may cause allergic reactions.[70] Phthalates are used to make plastics soft and flexible, but they leach out of the plastics and attach to dust particles that can be inhaled or ingested.[71] Children exposed to high levels of phthalates in household dust have been shown to be more likely to have asthma, eczema, and rhinitis than children exposed to low levels in previous studies.[72] Some studies suggest that phthalates may potentiate the immune response to other allergens.[73] Besides phthalates, other chemicals from plastics may also have adverse effects on the respiratory system, allergic airway inflammation, and the skin.[74] Overall, EDCs may interact with temperature and other environmental factors and can cause synergistic or antagonistic effects on immune systems.[75]

Impacts on Socioeconomic Status

CC is intertwined with SES in that poorer, historically minoritized populations are more impacted and its effects are a serious threat to socioeconomic stability, impacting the business community, and creating environmental injustice. Unfortunately, CC affects different regions and groups unevenly contributing to economic inequality between and within countries.[76] Across the globe, wealthy countries in colder regions may benefit long-term from warmer temperatures, while poor countries in hotter regions may have suffered from reduced agricultural productivity, water scarcity, and health risks.[77] However, given the interconnectedness of the global economy, adverse impacts will be experienced by all countries. The effects of redlining in the United States, segregation, and lack of resources in poorer communities will likely disproportionately limit access to potentially lifesaving resources, such as air conditioning during heat waves. The poorest and most marginalized people are often the most vulnerable to climate impacts, yet they have the least responsibility for causing them and fewer resources to address CC.[78]

SES as a measure of one's access to economic and social resources, such as income, education, and health care, can greatly influence the risk of developing allergies.[79] Low SES does not directly cause disease but is a correlate of factors that predict poorer health, such as access to health care, heat/air conditioning, local pollution levels, and access to healthy foods. Because low SES is associated with greater exposure to environmental pollutants, poor housing conditions, lack of preventive health care, and limited access to healthy foods, as well as with CC effects, the impacts of allergic diseases are disproportionately borne by low SES communities.[80]

Impacts on Gut Microbiota

CC can further affect gut microbiota, which is increasingly found to be associated with immune function.[81] Rising temperatures may alter the composition and diversity of microbial communities in the gut, leading to changes in metabolic functions and immune responses.[82] Additionally, CC could increase the exposure to environmental toxins that are released by pathogens.[83] Excessive antibiotic use can disrupt the balance of gut microbiota, altering the risk of disease associated with the gut microbiome.[83] Rising temperatures increase the spread of infectious diseases by expanding the range of disease vectors, such as mosquitoes and ticks, which increase the demand for antibiotics.[84] CC can also affect the behavior and distribution of animals that carry zoonotic diseases, such as rabies and anthrax, which again may require antibiotic or antiviral treatment.[85] CC may increase the contamination of water and soil by antibiotic residues from human and animal waste that may pose a risk for environmental and human health. Antibiotic residues can disrupt the balance of microbes in the environment and in the body, which may affect the immune system's ability to respond to allergens and infections.[86]

Impacts on Vulnerable Populations

CC and EC will influence subgroups of populations differently across the world with the elderly, children, pregnant women, and low-income communities facing higher risks for adverse health effects.[87] This is due to a combination of factors, such as their location, occupation, SES, education level, race and ethnicity, and age. These groups may have higher rates of existing medical conditions, such as asthma, diabetes, hypertension, and chronic obstructive pulmonary disease that can be exacerbated by CC and EC impacts. A study in Sweden by Schyllert and colleagues (2020) reported an interaction between income and sex in which women with low income had an increased risk for allergic asthma.[88] It is important to note that such results may not be generalizable to other populations and further studies are needed.

Strategies to Mitigate the Adverse Consequences of Exposome Change Due to Climate Change

Unfortunately, CC will not be alleviated in the short term, and to cope with these impacts, individuals and populations need to take action to protect themselves from EC by reducing their exposure to environmental triggers, enhancing their resilience through lifestyle modifications, and seeking timely medical attention when needed. Individuals with resources should adapt their lifestyle by adopting behaviors to reduce the impact of CC (eg, air conditioning, use of apps that predict weather and air pollution) in conjunctions with more sustainable practices, such as using renewable energy sources, public transport, and reduced fossil fuel use (eg, flying less). *Most importantly, policymakers must consider the needs of vulnerable populations to create programs to help them mitigate the risks of heat waves and other weather disasters that are specific to their communities as the impacts of CC are highly variable geographically.* This need is urgent. Populations also may need to reduce their waste and emissions, promote green spaces and urban planning, and enhance disaster preparedness. Such activities will increase resilience and support local communities and vulnerable subgroups of the population.

SUMMARY

As summarized herein, CC is part of the exposome and has both direct and indirect effects on environmental exposures and human health. Through a number of interconnected pathways, CC can have significant effects on the onset of allergies and related respiratory disorders and may pose a challenge for allergic individuals by enhancing propensity to exacerbation of their existing allergies. EC can have particular impacts on vulnerable populations, such as the elderly, children, or pregnant women, who may have weaker immune systems, higher sensitivity, or lower access to resources. Individuals and populations need to take action to protect themselves from EC, such as by reducing their exposure, enhancing their resilience, or advocating for policies that mitigate environmental hazards.

CLINICS CARE POINTS

- A comprehensive assessment of the patient's exposome history, including personal, occupational, and environmental factors, can help more comprehensively identify potential triggers and risk factors for allergic diseases
- A personalized approach to allergy management, taking into account the patient's exposome profile, genetic predisposition, comorbidities, and preferences, can improve outcomes and quality of life

DISCLOSURE

The authors have nothing to disclose.

ACKNOWLEDGMENT

The authors acknowledge financial support by the US National Institute of Health (grant numbers: P30ES023515 and UL1TR004419).

REFERENCES

1. Dessai S, Adger WN, Hulme M, et al. Defining and experiencing dangerous climate change. Climatic Change 2004;64:11–25.
2. Meinshausen M, Smith SJ, Calvin K, et al. The RCP greenhouse gas concentrations and their extensions from 1765 to 2300. Climatic Change 2011;109:213–41.
3. Kendon M, McCarthy M, Jevrejeva S, et al. State of the UK Climate 2020. Int J Climatol 2021;41:1–76.
4. Wild CP. The exposome: from concept to utility. Int J Epidemiol 2012;41(1):24–32.
5. Wright RO. Nature versus nurture—on the origins of a specious argument. Exposome 2022;2(1):osac005.

6. Vermeulen R, Schymanski EL, Barabási A-L, et al. The exposome and health: Where chemistry meets biology. Science 2020;367(6476):392–6.
7. Knol EF and Gilles S. Allergy: Type I, II, III, and IV, In: Michel MC, editor. *Allergic diseases–from basic mechanisms to comprehensive management and prevention*, 2021, Springer, 31–41. https://www.springer.com/series/164.
8. Katz DS, Baptist AP, Batterman SA. Modeling airborne pollen concentrations at an urban scale with pollen release from individual trees. Aerobiologia 2023;1–13.
9. D'Amato G, Chong-Neto HJ, Monge Ortega OP, et al. The effects of climate change on respiratory allergy and asthma induced by pollen and mold allergens. Allergy 2020;75(9):2219–28.
10. Clark S, Long AA, Gaeta TJ, et al. Multicenter study of emergency department visits for insect sting allergies. Journal of allergy and clinical immunology 2005; 116(3):643–9.
11. Pawankar R. Allergic diseases and asthma: a global public health concern and a call to action. BioMed Central 2014;7:1–3.
12. Hay RJ, Johns NE, Williams HC, et al. The Global Burden of Skin Disease in 2010: An Analysis of the Prevalence and Impact of Skin Conditions. J Invest Dermatol 2014;134(6):1527–34.
13. Zablotsky B, Black LI, Akinbami LJ. Diagnosed Allergic Conditions in Children Aged 0–17 Years. United States 2023;2021. https://www.cdc.gov/nchs/products/databriefs/db460.htm.
14. Dierick BJ, van der Molen T, Flokstra-de Blok BM, et al. Burden and socioeconomics of asthma, allergic rhinitis, atopic dermatitis and food allergy. Expert Rev Pharmacoecon Outcomes Res 2020;20(5):437–53.
15. Vazquez-Ortiz M, Angier E, Blumchen K, et al. Understanding the challenges faced by adolescents and young adults with allergic conditions: a systematic review. Allergy 2020;75(8):1850–80.
16. Jarosz M, Syed S, Błachut M, et al. Emotional distress and quality of life in allergic diseases. Wiad Lek 2020;73(2):370–3.
17. Masson-Delmotte V, Zhai P, Pörtner H-O, et al. Global warming of 1.5° C: IPCC special Report on impacts of global warming of 1.5° C above pre-industrial levels in Context of Strengthening response to climate change, sustainable Development, and Efforts to Eradicate, Poverty. Cambridge University Press; 2022. https://dlib.hust.edu.vn/handle/HUST/21737.
18. Requia WJ, Vicedo-Cabrera AM, de Schrijver E, et al. Association of high ambient temperature with daily hospitalization for cardiorespiratory diseases in Brazil: A national time-series study between 2008 and 2018. Environmental Pollution 2023;331:121851.
19. Requia WJ, Vicedo-Cabrera AM, de Schrijver E, et al. Low ambient temperature and hospitalization for cardiorespiratory diseases in Brazil. Environ Res 2023; 231:116231.
20. Williams K, Copsey D, Blockley E, et al. The Met Office global coupled model 3.0 and 3.1 (GC3. 0 and GC3. 1) configurations. J Adv Model Earth Syst 2018;10(2): 357–80.
21. Ebi KL, Capon A, Berry P, et al. Hot weather and heat extremes: health risks. The lancet 2021;398(10301):698–708.
22. Henderson SB, Brauer M, MacNab YC, et al. Three measures of forest fire smoke exposure and their associations with respiratory and cardiovascular health outcomes in a population-based cohort. Environmental health perspectives 2011; 119(9):1266–71.

23. Amini H, Nhung NTT, Schindler C, et al. Short-term associations between daily mortality and ambient particulate matter, nitrogen dioxide, and the air quality index in a Middle Eastern megacity. Environmental Pollution 2019;254:113121.
24. Amini H, Dehlendorff C, Lim Y-H, et al. Long-term exposure to air pollution and stroke incidence: A Danish Nurse cohort study. Environ Int 2020;142:105891.
25. Nhung NTT, Amini H, Schindler C, et al. Short-term association between ambient air pollution and pneumonia in children: A systematic review and meta-analysis of time-series and case-crossover studies. Environmental Pollution 2017;230: 1000–8.
26. Heydarpour P, Amini H, Khoshkish S, et al. Potential impact of air pollution on multiple sclerosis in Tehran, Iran. Neuroepidemiology 2015;43(3–4):233–8.
27. Xu R, Rahmandad H, Gupta M, et al. Weather, air pollution, and SARS-CoV-2 transmission: a global analysis. Lancet Planet Health 2021;5(10):e671–80.
28. Hong C, Mueller ND, Burney JA, et al. Impacts of ozone and climate change on yields of perennial crops in California. Nature Food 2020;1(3):166–72.
29. Jhun I, Coull BA, Schwartz J, et al. The impact of weather changes on air quality and health in the United States in 1994–2012. Environ Res Lett 2015;10(8): 084009.
30. Dupuy J-l, Fargeon H, Martin-StPaul N, et al. Climate change impact on future wildfire danger and activity in southern Europe: a review. Ann For Sci 2020; 77:1–24.
31. Naeher LP, Brauer M, Lipsett M, et al. Woodsmoke health effects: a review. Inhal Toxicol 2007;19(1):67–106.
32. Reid CE, Brauer M, Johnston FH, et al. Critical review of health impacts of wildfire smoke exposure. Environmental health perspectives 2016;124(9):1334–43.
33. Ziska L, Knowlton K, Rogers C, et al. Recent warming by latitude associated with increased length of ragweed pollen season in central North America. Proc Natl Acad Sci U S A 2011;108(10):4248–51.
34. Wayne P, Foster S, Connolly J, et al. Production of allergenic pollen by ragweed (Ambrosia artemisiifolia L.) is increased in CO2-enriched atmospheres. Ann Allergy Asthma Immunol 2002;88(3):279–82.
35. Beggs PJ, Clot B, Sofiev M, et al. Climate change, airborne allergens, and three translational mitigation approaches. EBioMedicine 2023;93:104478.
36. D'Amato G, Akdis C. Global warming, climate change, air pollution and allergies. Allergy 2020;75(9):2158–60.
37. Lam HC, Jarvis D, Fuertes E. Interactive effects of allergens and air pollution on respiratory health: a systematic review. Sci Total Environ 2021;757:143924.
38. Schramm P, Brown C, Saha S, et al. A systematic review of the effects of temperature and precipitation on pollen concentrations and season timing, and implications for human health. International journal of biometeorology 2021;65:1615–28.
39. Shea KM, Truckner RT, Weber RW, et al. Climate change and allergic disease. J Allergy Clin Immunol 2008;122(3):443–53 [quiz: 454–5].
40. D'Amato G, Vitale C, Sanduzzi A, et al. Allergenic pollen and pollen allergy in Europe. Allergy and Allergen Immunotherapy 2017;287–306.
41. Acevedo N, Zakzuk J, Caraballo L. House dust mite allergy under changing environments. Allergy, asthma & immunology research 2019;11(4):450–69.
42. Groot J, Tange Nielsen E, Fuhr Nielsen T, et al. Exposure to residential mold and dampness and the associations with respiratory tract infections and symptoms thereof in children in high income countries: A systematic review and meta-analyses of epidemiological studies. Paediatr Respir Rev 2023. https://doi.org/10.1016/j.prrv.2023.06.003.

43. Luschkova D, Traidl-Hoffmann C, Ludwig A. Climate change and allergies. Allergo Journal International 2022;31(4):114–20.
44. Suzuki N, Mittler R. Reactive oxygen species and temperature stresses: a delicate balance between signaling and destruction. Physiol Plantarum 2006; 126(1):45–51.
45. Gisler A. Allergies in urban areas on the rise: the combined effect of air pollution and pollen. Int J Publ Health 2021;42.
46. Pan Z, Dai Y, Akar-Ghibril N, et al. Impact of Air Pollution on Atopic Dermatitis: A Comprehensive Review. Clin Rev Allergy Immunol 2023;1–15.
47. Bellinato F, Adami G, Vaienti S, et al. Association between short-term exposure to environmental air pollution and psoriasis flare. JAMA dermatology 2022;158(4): 375–81.
48. Lowe ME, Akhtari FS, Potter TA, et al. The skin is no barrier to mixtures: Air pollutant mixtures and reported psoriasis or eczema in the Personalized Environment and Genes Study (PEGS). J Expo Sci Environ Epidemiol 2022;1–8.
49. Berger M, Bastl M, Bouchal J, et al. The influence of air pollution on pollen allergy sufferers. Allergologie Select 2021;5:345.
50. Mousavi SE, Amini H, Heydarpour P, et al. Air pollution, environmental chemicals, and smoking may trigger vitamin D deficiency: Evidence and potential mechanisms. Environ Int 2019;122:67–90.
51. Sangüesa J, Sunyer J, Garcia-Esteban R, et al. Prenatal and child vitamin D levels and allergy and asthma in childhood. Pediatr Res 2023;93(6):1745–51.
52. Johansson O. Disturbance of the immune system by electromagnetic fields—A potentially underlying cause for cellular damage and tissue repair reduction which could lead to disease and impairment. Pathophysiology 2009;16(2–3): 157–77.
53. Stein Y, Udasin IG. Electromagnetic hypersensitivity (EHS, microwave syndrome)–Review of mechanisms. Environ Res 2020;186:109445.
54. Belpomme D, Irigaray P. Why electrohypersensitivity and related symptoms are caused by non-ionizing man-made electromagnetic fields: An overview and medical assessment. Environ Res 2022;212:113374.
55. Vicente JL. Climate change and the effects on environment and exposure to chemicals. Eur J Publ Health 2021;31(Supplement_3). ckab164. 267.
56. Wickland KP, Waldrop MP, Aiken GR, et al. Dissolved organic carbon and nitrogen release from boreal Holocene permafrost and seasonally frozen soils of Alaska. Environ Res Lett 2018;13(6):065011.
57. Pettoello-Mantovani M, Indrio F, Francavilla R, et al. The effects of climate change and exposure to endocrine disrupting chemicals on children's health: a challenge for pediatricians. Global Pediatrics 2023;100047.
58. Monneret C. What is an endocrine disruptor? Comptes Rendus Biol 2017; 340(9–10):403–5.
59. Kabir ER, Rahman MS, Rahman I. A review on endocrine disruptors and their possible impacts on human health. Environ Toxicol Pharmacol 2015;40(1): 241–58.
60. Schug TT, Janesick A, Blumberg B, et al. Endocrine disrupting chemicals and disease susceptibility. J Steroid Biochem Mol Biol 2011;127(3–5):204–15.
61. Zhu L, Jiang C, Panthi S, et al. Impact of high precipitation and temperature events on the distribution of emerging contaminants in surface water in the Mid-Atlantic, United States. Sci Total Environ 2021;755:142552.

62. Cestonaro LV, Macedo SMD, Piton YV, et al. Toxic effects of pesticides on cellular and humoral immunity: an overview. Immunopharmacol Immunotoxicol 2022; 44(6):816–31.
63. Loffredo LF, Coden ME, Berdnikovs S. Endocrine disruptor bisphenol A (BPA) triggers systemic para-inflammation and is sufficient to induce airway allergic sensitization in mice. Nutrients 2020;12(2):343.
64. Gusev EY, Zotova NV. Cellular stress and general pathological processes. Curr Pharmaceut Des 2019;25(3):251–97.
65. Thaiss CA, Levy M, Grosheva I, et al. Hyperglycemia drives intestinal barrier dysfunction and risk for enteric infection. Science 2018;359(6382):1376–83.
66. Robinson DS. Regulatory T cells and asthma. Clin Exp Allergy 2009;39(9): 1314–23.
67. Yang Y, Guo Y, O'Brien AM, et al. Biological Responses to Climate Change and Nanoplastics Are Altered in Concert: Full-Factor Screening Reveals Effects of Multiple Stressors on Primary Producers. Environmental Science & Technology 2020;54(4):2401–10.
68. Hu L, Fu J, Wang S, et al. Microplastics generated under simulated fire scenarios: characteristics, antimony leaching, and toxicity. Environmental Pollution 2021; 269:115905.
69. Alabi OA, Ologbonjaye KI, Awosolu O, et al. Public and environmental health effects of plastic wastes disposal: a review. J Toxicol Risk Assess 2019; 5(021):1–13.
70. Zhang Y, Lyu L, Tao Y, et al. Health risks of phthalates: A review of immunotoxicity. Environmental Pollution 2022;120173.
71. Sireli UT, Filazi A, Yurdakok-Dikmen B, et al. Determination of phthalate residues in different types of yogurt by gas chromatography-mass spectrometry and estimation of yogurt-related intake of phthalates. Food Anal Methods 2017;10: 3052–62.
72. Bornehag C-G, Nanberg E. Phthalate exposure and asthma in children. Int J Androl 2010;33(2):333–45.
73. Kimber I, Dearman RJ. An assessment of the ability of phthalates to influence immune and allergic responses. Toxicology 2010;271(3):73–82.
74. Kozioł M, Krasa A, Łopuszyńska AM, et al. The influence of bisphenol A on the human body. Journal of Education, Health and Sport 2021;11(9):238–45.
75. Hamid N, Junaid M, Pei D-S. Combined toxicity of endocrine-disrupting chemicals: A review. Ecotoxicol Environ Saf 2021;215:112136.
76. Rao ND, Min J. Less global inequality can improve climate outcomes. Wiley Interdisciplinary Reviews: Clim Change 2018;9(2):e513.
77. Mendelsohn R, Dinar A, Williams L. The distributional impact of climate change on rich and poor countries. Environ Dev Econ 2006;11(2):159–78.
78. Newell P, Srivastava S, Naess LO, et al. Toward transformative climate justice: An emerging research agenda. Wiley Interdisciplinary Reviews: Clim Change 2021; 12(6):e733.
79. Kim J, Kim B, Kim DH, et al. In Association between Socioeconomic Status and Healthcare utilization for children with allergic Diseases: Korean National Health and Nutritional Examination Survey (2015–2019). Healthcare 2023;2023:492.
80. Kojima R, Shinohara R, Kushima M, et al. Association between Household Income and Allergy Development in Children: The Japan Environment and Children's Study. Int Arch Allergy Immunol 2022;183(2):201–9.
81. Williams CE, Williams CL, Logan ML. Climate change is not just global warming: Multidimensional impacts on animal gut microbiota. Microb Biotechnol 2023.

82. Sepulveda J, Moeller AH. The effects of temperature on animal gut microbiomes. Front Microbiol 2020;11:384.
83. Boxall AB, Hardy A, Beulke S, et al. Impacts of climate change on indirect human exposure to pathogens and chemicals from agriculture. Environmental health perspectives 2009;117(4):508–14.
84. Edelson PJ, Harold R, Ackelsberg J, et al. Climate change and the epidemiology of infectious diseases in the United States. Clin Infect Dis 2023;76(5):950–6.
85. Cao B, Bai C, Wu K, et al. Tracing the future of epidemics: Coincident niche distribution of host animals and disease incidence revealed climate-correlated risk shifts of main zoonotic diseases in China. Global Change Biol 2023.
86. Duan Y, Chen Z, Tan L, et al. Gut resistomes, microbiota and antibiotic residues in Chinese patients undergoing antibiotic administration and healthy individuals. Sci Total Environ 2020;705:135674.
87. Astone R, Vaalavuo M. Climate change and health: Consequences of high temperatures among vulnerable groups in Finland. International Journal of Social Determinants of Health and Health Services 2023;53(1):94–111.
88. Schyllert C, Lindberg A, Hedman L, et al. Low socioeconomic status relates to asthma and wheeze, especially in women. ERJ open research 2020;6(3).

Respiratory Health Effects of Air Pollutants

David B. Peden, MD, MS

KEYWORDS

• Air pollution • PM2.5 • Asthma • Pneumonia • COVID-19

KEY POINTS

• Air pollution induces and exacerbates asthma.
• Air pollution increases risk for infection.
• Particulate matter between 0.5 and 2.5 microns in diameter is a significant cause of asthma and infection.
• Pollutants augment response to allergens.
• Persons with asthma have increased responsiveness to pollutants.

INTRODUCTION

Environmental air pollutants are a significant cause for development and exacerbation of respiratory disease.[1–3] This chapter focuses on respiratory health effects of pollutants in asthma and lower airway respiratory infections, a common cause for asthma exacerbation. This review covers epidemiologic studies assessing the exacerbations or development of respiratory disorders, interplay between pollution exposure and immunoglobulin E (IgE)-mediated responses, risk factors that may affect pollutant related respiratory diseases, and mechanistic and controlled exposure studies that provide physiologic plausibility for health effects of these pollutants. This chapter also highlights examples of potential personal and policy interventions to address pollutant-induced respiratory disease.

The respiratory diseases most clearly affected by air pollution are asthma, lower respiratory tract infections (LRTI), and chronic obstructive pulmonary disease (COPD).[4] As will be detailed later, exacerbation of asthma is clearly linked to increased levels of ambient air pollutants, usually with a 24- to 72-hour lag time.[1] There is a growing body of evidence that genesis of asthma is also linked to pollutant exposure, especially perinatal exposures.[3,4] Acute pollutant exposures are also linked to episodes of LRTI.[4] It is less clear if ambient air pollution affects development of COPD, but

Division of Pediatric Allergy & Immunology and, Center for Environmental Medicine, Asthma and Lung Biology, The School of Medicine, The University of North Carolina at Chapel Hill, UNC School of Medicine, 104 Mason Farm Road, CB#7310, Chapel Hill, NC 27599-7310, USA
E-mail address: peden@med.unc.edu

Immunol Allergy Clin N Am 44 (2024) 15–33
https://doi.org/10.1016/j.iac.2023.07.004
0889-8561/24/© 2023 Elsevier Inc. All rights reserved.
immunology.theclinics.com

pollutant exposure may certainly cause exacerbation of this disorder, and COPD has the highest mortality rate associated with air pollutant exposure.[5]

Among the air pollutants most associated with adverse health outcomes are ozone (O3) and particulate matter (PM) between 0.5 and 2.5 microns in diameter (PM2.5) or between 2.5 and 10 microns in diameter (PM10). Other pollutants include SO2, oxides of nitrogen (NOx), and lead. In the United States, the Clean Air Act requires the United States Environmental Protection Agency (EPA) to regulate air quality to levels codified by the National Ambient Air Quality Standards (NAAQS, **Table 1**).[1] As stated by the EPA, the primary NAAQS standards are established for public health protection, which specifically include the health of persons with asthma, children, and elderly people and other "sensitive" populations. The NAAQS secondary standards are set to protect against decreased visibility and damage to animals, crops, vegetation, and buildings.

Climate change and air pollution are intertwined, as previously reviewed.[6,7] This interrelationship is depicted in **Fig. 1** from a review by Pacheco and colleagues.[6] Fossil fuel use generates pollutants that cause climate change including the greenhouse gases carbon dioxide and methane. Conversely, climate change enhances production

Table 1
National ambient air quality standards.

Pollutant [links to historical tables of NAAQS reviews]		Primary/ Secondary	Averaging Time	Level	Form
Carbon Monoxide (CO)		primary	8 hours	9 ppm	Not to be exceeded more than once per year
			1 hour	35 ppm	
Lead (Pb)		primary and secondary	Rolling 3 month average	0.15 µg/m³	Not to be exceeded
Nitrogen Dioxide (NO₂)		primary	1 hour	100 ppb	98th percentile of 1-hour daily maximum concentrations, averaged over 3 years
		primary and secondary	1 year	53 ppb	Annual Mean
Ozone (O₃)		primary and secondary	8 hours	0.070 ppm	Annual fourth-highest daily maximum 8-hour concentration, averaged over 3 years
Particle Pollution (PM)	PM₂.₅	primary	1 year	12.0 µg/m³	annual mean, averaged over 3 years
		secondary	1 year	15.0 µg/m³	annual mean, averaged over 3 years
		primary and secondary	24 hours	35 µg/m³	98th percentile, averaged over 3 years
	PM₁₀	primary and secondary	24 hours	150 µg/m³	Not to be exceeded more than once per year on average over 3 years
Sulfur Dioxide (SO₂)		primary	1 hour	75 ppb	99th percentile of 1-hour daily maximum concentrations, averaged over 3 years
		secondary	3 hours	0.5 ppm	Not to be exceeded more than once per year

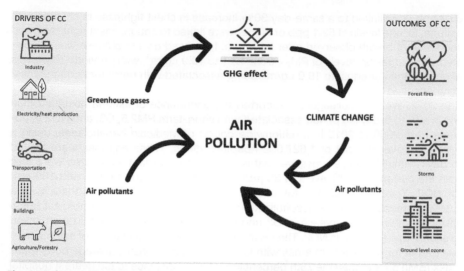

Fig. 1. Relationship between the drivers of climate change (CC) and the outcomes of CC and air pollution. (*From* Pacheco SE, Guidos-Fogelbach G, Annesi-Maesano I, et al. Climate change and global issues in allergy and immunology. *J Allergy Clin Immunol*. Dec 2021;148(6):1366-1377. https://doi.org/10.1016/j.jaci.2021.10.01.)

of ambient air pollutants. Warmer atmospheres will result in more heat inversions that result in stagnant air containing oxides of nitrogen and volatile organic compounds that interact with ultraviolet light, resulting in O3 generation. Warmer climates also promote increased occurrence of wildfires with increased levels of PM2.5. In addition, warming conditions have already been shown to cause earlier and longer pollination seasons, enhancing airborne allergen exposure.[8-11] In studies of ragweed, oak, and birch, exposure of plants to air pollutants cause both increased allergen levels and allergenicity in pollen.[8,12,13] Taken together, air pollution contributes to climate change, which worsens air pollution, with both phenomena inducing increased ambient air pollen exposures.[14] These exposures contribute to exacerbation of airway diseases.

DISCUSSION
Asthma

It has been well established that persons with asthma have increased susceptibility to adverse health outcomes associated with pollutant exposure.[1,2] Ozone is perhaps the most encountered pollutant associated with asthma events, although PM2.5, NO2, SO2, and traffic-related air pollutants (TRAPs) have all been linked to increased occurrences of asthma. Environmental endotoxin has also been associated with exacerbation of asthma[15-17] and is a component of airborne PM.[18,19] Numerous epidemiology studies across decades demonstrate that emergency room visits, hospitalizations, and even asthma mortality are increased following pollutant exposure. Although it is well established that asthma events are linked to exposures higher than established NAAQS levels for pollutants, there is concern that levels of air pollution less than NAAQS levels also induce exacerbations of asthma.

In 2003, Gent and colleagues[20] reported the effect of ambient air pollutants in 271 children from a cohort of families living in Connecticut and the Springfield area of Massachusetts. They reported that 8-hour average levels of ozone higher than or equal to

63.3 ppb were linked to a same-day 30% increase in chest tightness in children with asthma. Ozone levels of 52.1 ppb or higher were linked to cough, chest tightness, and shortness of breath observed after 24 hours. Increased chest tightness was associated with same-day levels of $PM_{2.5}$ from 12.1 to 18.9 $\mu g/m^3$, with previous-day levels of greater than or equal to 19.0 $\mu g/m^3$ being associated with persistent cough, chest tightness, and shortness of breath.

In 2022, Wei and colleagues[21] reported the occurrence of asthma hospitalization within a 0- to 6-day lag period associated with short-term PM2.5, O3, and NO2 exposures from 2000 to 2012 in a nationwide cohort of Medicaid beneficiaries, using a case-crossover dataset of 1,627,002 hospitalizations. These analyses were limited to days within the case-crossover dataset in which pollutant exposures were less than the current NAAQS levels of 35 $\mu g/m3$ for PM2.5, 70 ppb for O3, and 100 ppb for NO2. They reported that for each 1 $\mu g/m3$ increase in PM2.5, there was a 0.31% increase in asthma hospitalization, with a 0.10% increase in hospitalization linked to each 1 ppb increase in O3 and a 0.28% increase in hospitalization linked to each 1-ppb increase in NO2. They also found significantly higher risk of asthma hospitalization for persons from areas with lower population density, average body mass index (BMI) greater than the 75th percentile, or longer distance to the nearest hospital for these pollutant exposures.

In a 2023 report, Bi and colleagues[22] examined 3.19 million emergency department (ED) visits from 2005 to 2014 across the United States for asthma associated with exposure to fine and coarse PM, major PM components, and gaseous pollutants. They assessed ED visit and air pollution data from 53 monitoring sites in 10 states. Using quasi-Poisson log-linear time-series models with unconstrained distributed exposure lags they estimated site-specific acute effects of air pollution on overall and age-stratified asthma ED visits. They observed positive associations between multiday exposure to all monitored pollutants and asthma ED visits. Across an 8-day lag period, they observed rate ratio increases in ED visits (with 95% confidence interval [CI]) by pollutant increase of 1.016 (1.008, 1.025) per each 6.3 μg increase in PM2.5, 1.014 (1.007, 1.020 95% CI) per each 9.6 μg increase in PM10, 1.008 (0.995, 1.022 95% CI) per 0.02 ppm increase in O3, and 1.016 (1.009, 1.024) per 2.8 μg increase in organic carbon. Although PM2.5 had strong effects across all ages and ozone had more impact on adults, most pollutant effects were more pronounced in children.

In another 2023 report, Altman and colleagues[23] undertook a secondary analysis of 2 pediatric cohorts, with analyses of 168 children aged 6 to 17 years from an observational study undertaken from 2015 to 2017 and 189 from a clinical trial of participants aged 6 to 20 years performed from 2006 to 2009. The investigators had air quality index values and air pollutant concentrations from across the time frame of these studies for PM2.5, PM10, O3, NO2, SO2, CO, and Pb from the US Environmental Protection Agency and were able to link these pollutant metrics to each exacerbation for each participant, focusing on nonviral related disease. They reported that air quality index values, especially increased PM2.5 and O3 concentrations, were significantly associated with asthma exacerbations and decreases in pulmonary function that occurred in those children without a viral infection (**Fig. 2**). Taken together, these reports indicate that pollutant exposure lower than current NAAQS levels trigger asthma exacerbations.

Although asthma exacerbations are clearly induced by pollutant exposure, there is a growing body of evidence that development of asthma is associated with ambient air pollutant exposure. One example of such data is from a 2015 study,[24] in which investigators recorded annual average air pollution concentrations of NO2, PM2.5, and PM10 and soot obtained at home addresses of a birth cohort of 14,126 participants

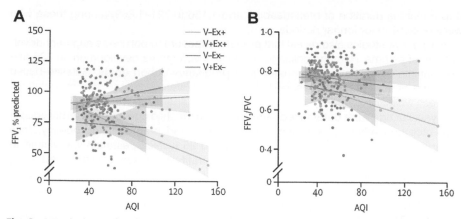

Fig. 2. Associations of pulmonary functions with AQI values. Associations of FEV1% predicted (*A*) and FEV1/FVC ratio (*B*) with AQI measured on the same day. Regression lines, 95% CIs, and all data points are shown for each group. There were 16 data points for the V–Ex + group, 36 data points for the V + Ex + group, 70 data points for the V–Ex– group, and 116 data points for the V + Ex– group. AQI, air quality index; FEV1% predicted, forced expiratory volume in 1 s as a percentage of predicted; FEV1/FVC, ratio of forced expiratory volume in 1 s to forced vital capacity; V–Ex+, nonviral event without exacerbation; V + Ex+, viral event with exacerbation; V–Ex–, nonviral event without exacerbation; V + Ex–, viral event without exacerbation. (*From* Altman MC, Kattan M, O'Connor GT, et al. Associations between outdoor air pollutants and non-viral asthma exacerbations and airway inflammatory responses in children and adolescents living in urban areas in the USA: a retrospective secondary analysis. *Lancet Planet Health.* Jan 2023;7(1):e33-e44. https://doi.org/10.1016/s2542-5196(22)00302-3.)

(derived from 4 prospective birth cohort studies from Germany, Sweden, and the Netherlands) to assess the impact of these exposures on asthma and rhinoconjunctivitis. This study had 14 to 16 years of follow-up, and researchers analyzed longitudinal associations of air pollution exposure at participants' birth addresses and addresses at the time of follow-up with asthma and rhinoconjunctivitis incidence and prevalence in cohort-specific analyses. They reported that the risk of incident asthma up to age 14 to 16 years increased with increasing exposure to NO2 (odds ratio 1.13 per 10 µg/m3 [95% CI 1·02–1·25]) and a PM2.5 absorbance, a measure of soot (odd ratio of 1.29 per 1 unit [95% CI 1·00–1·66]) at the birth address. These associations with asthma were more consistent after age 4 years than before that age.

In a 2021 report, Zhang and colleagues[25] undertook a cross-sectional survey of 5788 preschool children aged 3 to 5 years in central China. Using machine learning–based spatiotemporal models, they assessed in utero and first-year exposures to ambient PM1 (PM with a mean diameter of ≤1 micron in diameter), PM2.5, and PM10 and performed a time-to-event analysis to examine associations between residential PM exposures and childhood onset of asthma and wheezing. They observed that early life size-specific PM exposures, particularly during pregnancy, were significantly associated with increased risk of asthma. They reported that for each 10 µg/m3 increase in in utero and first-year PM1 exposure there was an asthma hazard ratio of 1.618 (95% CI, 1.159–2.258; *P* = .005) and 1.543 (0.822–2.896; *P* = .177), respectively. Duration of breast feeding also was a risk modifier for pollutant-induced asthma, with each 10 µg/m3 increase in in utero exposure to PM1 being associated with a hazard ratio of 2.260 (1.393–3.666) among children with

0 to 5 months duration of breastfeeding and 1.156 (0.721–1.853) among those who were breast-fed for longer periods.

Prospective studies also reveal that prenatal exposure to pollutants augment development of asthma. Hsu and colleagues[26] examined asthma development in 736 full-term infants born to women enrolled in a pregnancy cohort study. Satellite-based estimates of daily PM2.5 exposure during gestation were assessed, and associations between weekly averaged gestational PM2.5 levels and physician-diagnosed asthma by 6 years of age were determined. After adjusting for child age, sex, maternal education, race and ethnicity, smoking, stress, atopy, and prepregnancy obesity, they observed that PM2.5 exposure between 16 and 25 weeks' gestation was linked to increased physician-diagnosed asthma. When stratifying by sex, only men had a significant relationship between prenatal PM2.5 and asthma development. In another study from this cohort by Bose and colleagues,[27] the effect of daily ambient air gestational nitrite exposure in 725 mother-child dyads on physician-diagnosed asthma was assessed. They observed that 2 periods of gestation (7–19 and 33–40 weeks) were associated with greater odds of developing asthma by age 6 years in boys born to women under high prenatal. The overall odd ratio (OR) for development of asthma was also significant (OR:2.64, 95% CI = 1.27–5.39; per interquartile range increase in ln nitrite). These prospective studies both show that prenatal pollutant exposures augment development of asthma in men.

In a 2020 report of an ATS workshop on the impact of outdoor ambient air pollution on lung disease, a review of the literature revealed a clear relationship between exposure to TRAPs and PM2.5 and incident asthma in children.[4] There are also reports of these pollutants being associated with incident asthma in adults, although these data are less compelling for adults than for children. There are also observations that ambient air ozone exposure is associated with incident asthma in children and adults. However, these data are not as robust as the data for TRAPs and PM2.5. All this said, the preponderance of evidence demonstrates that prolonged exposure to ambient air pollutants, especially TRAPs and PM2.5, contributes to childhood incident asthma.

There are also emerging data that indicate that ambient air pollution exposure contributes to development of allergic disease, which is a major risk factor for development of childhood asthma. Several animal studies show that experimental perinatal exposure to pollutants enhances IgE sensitization to allergens.[4] In human experimental studies, challenge with diesel exhaust particles was shown to skew immune response toward T2 responses, including nasal immunization to keyhole limpet hemocyanin, showing human proof of concept that pollutant exposure can promote T2 responses to antigens.[28–30] These studies are consistent with several epidemiologic studies that demonstrate that early life and perinatal exposure to air pollutants are associated with development of atopy, as reviewed by Burbank and colleagues.[31]

Exacerbation of asthma due to pollutant exposure may occur because persons with asthma may have increased susceptibility to air pollutant effects or because air pollutants enhance T2 inflammatory responses to allergen. Acute increases in inflammation are a central component of asthma exacerbation. Controlled exposure studies involving challenge with a pollutant have been used to define airway inflammatory responses to pollutants and have been used to compare responses of volunteers with asthma with those without asthma.[1]

Scannell and colleagues[32] reported that persons with asthma had enhanced neutrophilic responses to ozone than did those without asthma using a controlled exposure protocol to 0.2 ppm O3 for 2 hours. Our group also examined the effect of 0.4 ppm for a 2-hour ozone exposure in persons with asthma and those without asthma.[33] We observed that after O3 challenge, when compared with healthy volunteers, atopic and atopic asthmatic subjects had increased sputum neutrophil numbers and interleukin-8 (IL-8) levels, with atopic asthmatic subjects having increased sputum IL-6 and IL-1β levels as well. In a subsequent evaluation of gene expression profiles recovered from sputum samples we found a marked difference in gene expression profiles, including increased expression of IL-6, IL-8, and IL-18 in asthmatics (**Fig. 3**).[34] Persons with asthma also have modestly increased neutrophilic inflammatory responses to woodsmoke particles[35] and concentrated air particulates.[36] Intriguingly, patients with asthma have decreased inflammatory response to inhaled endotoxin (a common component of PM) when compared with healthy volunteers.[37]

We and other investigators have also examined the effect of pollutant challenge on T2 responses to pollutants. Ozone has been reported to induce eosinophilic responses in the upper[38,39] and bronchial airways[40] of persons with allergic asthma. Pollutants may decrease the provocative dose of allergen required to elicit a 15% or 20% decrease in FEV1 (the allergen PD15 or PD20). One study has shown that combined exposure to sulfur dioxide and nitrogen dioxide have been reported to enhance spirometric response to inhaled allergen.[41] Low-level endotoxin challenge also has been reported to lower the PD20 of allergen in allergic asthmatics.[42] Studies of the effect of ozone on immediate bronchospastic responses to inhaled allergens have been mixed, with some studies demonstrating an enhancement of allergen reactivity, others suggesting that perhaps subgroups of allergic persons have increased allergen responses following ozone exposure, with other studies using shorter-term low-level ozone exposures showing no enhancement of response to allergen.[43-47] However, overall, ozone likely enhances allergen responses in at least some allergic asthmatics.

Several studies reveal that pollutants enhance allergen-induced airway inflammation. In the nasal airways of allergic persons, ozone exposure enhances allergen-induced eosinophilic inflammation.[38] Endotoxin challenge has been shown to enhance eosinophilic responses to allergen in the nasal[48] and bronchial[49] airways of allergic asthmatics. Diesel exhaust exposure also enhances allergen-induced inflammatory biomarkers in the lower airway.[50] Taken together, these studies demonstrate that pollutants augment response to allergen in allergic persons, although this effect is variable and may depend on yet unidentified risk factors in a subset of exposure persons. The impact of pollutants on response to allergen takes on added importance with climate change, which drives increases in both pollutant and ambient air allergen levels.

Pollutant Exposures and Respiratory Infection

Pneumonia and bronchitis are common clinical conditions that are modified by pollutant exposure. Epidemiologic studies provide the most robust evidence of the effects of pollutants on viral infection. In 2018, Horne and colleagues[51] used an observational case-crossover design of 146,397 persons living on the Wasatch Front in Utah who had an acute lower respiratory infection (ALRI) diagnosis. They assessed PM2.5 levels using community-based air quality monitors obtained between 1999 and 2016 and determined the odds ratios for ALRI health care encounters stratified by age (0–2, 3–17, and >18 years). Most of those with ALRI were 0 to 2 years of age (112,467, 77%), with a cumulative 28-day OR of 1.15/10 µg/m3 (95% CI, 1.12–1.19), with a similar OR for older children as well. It was noted that laboratory-confirmed respiratory syncytial virus and influenza cases increased following elevated ambient PM2.5 levels. Persons who were overweight, employed, or smokers had increased effects of pollutants.

Liu and colleagues[52] examined the relationship between air pollution and pneumonia in a cohort of 325,367 participants from multicenter project ELAPSE (Effects of Low-Level Air Pollution: A Study in Europe) across 6 European nations. Within

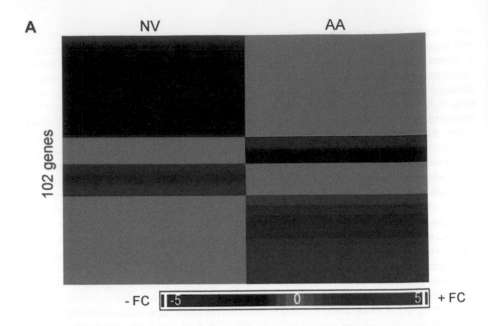

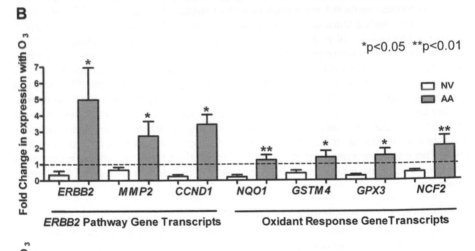

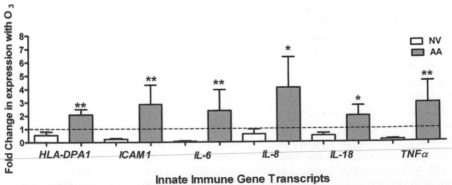

Fig. 3. O3-induced transcript profiles in healthy volunteers (NV) and AAs. (*A*) Heat map of O3-modulated genes in HVs and AAs with low (*blue*) and high (*red*) expression. (*B*) Changes

this cohort, 712 died of pneumonia and influenza combined, 682 from pneumonia, and 695 from ALRI. Exposure to NO2 and black carbon (BC) were linked to 10% to 12% increase in mortality from pneumonia and influenza. However, the hazard ratio was 1.12/10 μg/m3 for NO2 (0.99–1.26 95% CI) and 1.10/0.5 μg/m3 for BC (0.97–1.24 95% CI), which represented a trend toward significance. Stronger associations between pollutant exposure and NO2 or BC were noted in persons who were overweight, smokers, or employed.

The COVID-19 pandemic provided a significant temporal natural experiment in assessing the effect of pollutant exposure on infection, with SARS-CoV2 being an exemplar pathogen. In one study, Bozack and colleagues[53] examined the role of long-term pollution exposure on COVID-19 infection outcomes in New York City from March 8, 2020 to August 30, 2020. They assessed mortality, intensive care unit (ICU) admission and intubation in 6542 people with positive SARS-CoV2 polymerase chain reaction tests. They estimated the annual average concentrations of PM2.5, NO2, and BC for each person's home address and assessed the relationship between these exposures and COVID-19 outcomes. Two thousand forty-four people died (31%), 1237 were admitted to the ICU (19%), and 1051 were intubated. Long-term PM2.5 exposure was associated with a risk ratio of 1.11/1 μg/m3 increase in PM2.5 for mortality (1.02–1.21 95% CI) and 1.13/1 μg/m3 increase in PM2.5 (1.00–1.28 95% CI), with no effect seen with NO2 or BC with no increased risk for intubation being observed.

The impact of short-term exposure to pollutants on COVID-19 outcomes has also been examined. Early in the pandemic, Yee and colleagues[54] undertook a meta-analysis of numerous studies assessing the relationship between short-term pollutant exposure and COVID-19 exposures. They reported that an increased effect of short-term exposure to air pollutants and pneumonia-specific hospital admission or emergency room visit, especially for PM and NO2. In a study by Xu and colleagues,[53] the relationship between COVID-19 infection outcomes and short-term exposure to PM2.5 and O3 was explored. They examined cases in 554 counties in the United States for PM2.5 and COVID-19 outcomes and 670 counties for O3 impacts on COVID-19 outcomes, which yielded 2.1 million cases from March 1 to June 30, 2020. They found that for each 10 μg/m^3 increase in PM2.5 the number of daily confirmed cases increases by 9.41% (CI: 8.77%–10.04%) for PM2.5 and by 2.42% (CI: 1.56%–3.28%) for O$_3$. More studies are described in a review by Sheppard and colleagues.[54–56] Collectively, these results indicate that short-term exposure to PM2.5 is an important factor in acquiring SARS-CoV2 infection (**Fig. 4**).

In reviews by Burbank,[57] Monoson and colleagues,[58] and Beentjes and colleagues,[59] several reports are assessed demonstrating a link between pollutants (especially PM2.5) and increased risk for infection. Children seem to be an especially susceptible group. Several potential mechanisms by which pollutants enhance risk for infection include impairment of innate immune cells, reduction in mucociliary clearance, and impaired barrier function of the airway epithelium as potential mechanisms by which pollutant exposure may affect response to respiratory pathogens. The

---

with O3 in the PCR-amplified ERBB2 pathway, oxidant response, and innate immune transcripts relative to beta-actin (n = 6 HVs and 8 AAs). Mean changes in gene expression with O3 (±SEMs) are shown. Nonparametric t tests (Mann-Whitney tests) were used to compare differences in HVs and AAs. (*From* Hernandez M, Brickey WJ, Alexis NE, et al. Airway cells from atopic asthmatic patients exposed to ozone display an enhanced innate immune gene profile. *J Allergy Clin Immunol.* 1/2012 2012;129(1):259-261.)

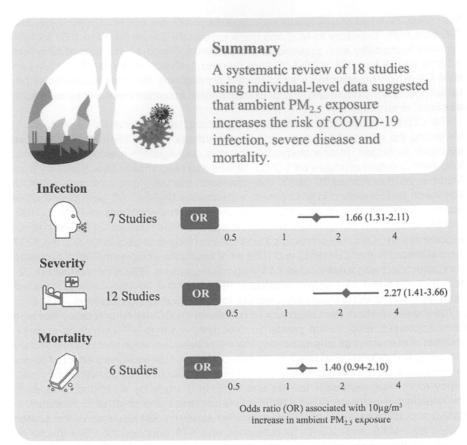

Summary

A systematic review of 18 studies using individual-level data suggested that ambient $PM_{2.5}$ exposure increases the risk of COVID-19 infection, severe disease and mortality.

Infection

7 Studies　OR　1.66 (1.31–2.11)

0.5　1　2　4

Severity

12 Studies　OR　2.27 (1.41–3.66)

0.5　1　2　4

Mortality

6 Studies　OR　1.40 (0.94–2.10)

0.5　1　2　4

Odds ratio (OR) associated with $10\mu g/m^3$ increase in ambient $PM_{2.5}$ exposure

Fig. 4. A systematic review of 18 studies using individual-level data suggested that ambient PM2.5 exposure increases the risk of COVID-19 infection, severe disease, and mortality. (*From* Sheppard et al, Sci Total Environ. 2023 Jul 1; 880: 163272. Published online 2023 Apr 7. https://doi.org/10.1016/j.scitotenv.2023.163272.)

impact of air pollutants on airway infection remains an underappreciated area of focus and is key to assessing the impact of pollution and climate on respiratory health.

Personal Interventions

The most well-accepted personal intervention to reduce the impact of air pollution on health is the use of appropriately fitted N95 masks, which filter greater than 95% of PM2.5 particulates present in the ambient atmosphere. These are recommended by NIOSH for occupational settings and require appropriate fit testing for optimal use. There are other face masks that can be used to reduce inhalation of particles from ambient air. Early in the COVID-19 pandemic, there was substantial interest in examining various face masks to determine if they might protect against inhalation of droplets contaminated by SARS-CoV2. In one study testing filtration effectiveness of various mask types, sodium chloride particles with a count median diameter of 0.05 μm (0.02–0.06 μm) were used, a size that is like that of PM2.5 pollutant particles (0.05–2.5 μm in diameter).[60] In these tests, a 3M 9210 NIOSH–approved N95 respirator had a mean fitted filtration efficiency (FFE) of 98.4%, compared with 71.5% for surgical mask with ties, 38.5% for a procedure mask with ear loops, and 49% for a folded "bandit" style bandana.

Kodros and colleagues[61] modeled the potential health protection from PM2.5/wildfire particle exposure by assessing FFE of various mask types in an in vitro laboratory setting and using these data in a mathematical model to assess potential health protection of various masks. They estimated that N95 respirators would reduce PM2.5 exposure by factor of 14, whereas synthetic fiber masks would reduce exposure by a factor of 2.2 to 4.2 and surgical masks would reduce exposure by a factor of 1.7. Using PM2.5 data from the 2012 Washington State fire season, they estimated that N95 and surgical masks might have reduced hospitalizations by 22% to 39% and 9% to 24%, respectively. To our review, masks have not been tested in a clinical study designed to assess reduction in adverse health outcome associated with PM2.5 outside of occupational settings. It seems reasonable that for persons at increased risk, using a mask with higher FFE would offer the most protection. However, this has not been tested in a randomized controlled trial as an intervention to reduce adverse health outcomes associated with PM2.5 exposure.

Use of high-efficiency particle accumulator (HEPA) filtration devices has also been suggested as a possible engineering approach to reduce PM2.5 exposure. These devices have been tested as part of a multimodal environmental intervention for children with asthma but was found to be important only in homes where smokers lived.[62] In one study of 43 children,[63] air filtration was associated with a mean 63.4% decrease in PM2.5 compared with sham filtration. There was no change in spirometry in these children, but there was improvement in lung mechanics, including a mean 24.4% reduction in total airway resistance and a 22.2% reduction in small airway resistance. There was also a 26.7% mean reduction in exhaled nitric oxide. As reviewed by Allen and Barn,[64] several randomized studies demonstrated substantial reduction in indoor PM2.5 levels. Air filtration was also associated with improved systemic blood pressure, endothelial function, and systemic inflammation. Although large-scale studies of air filtration for asthma are lacking, available evidence suggests that air filtration may be helpful for reducing PM2.5 and improving health outcomes.

Pharmacologic interventions have been proposed as interventions to prevent adverse effects related to air pollution. In controlled exposure studies, Vagaggini and colleagues[65] demonstrated that both inhaled budesonide and prednisone inhibited ozone-induced inflammation without affecting the spirometric response to ozone. Holz and colleagues[66] and Alexis and colleagues[67] made similar observations with fluticasone treatment. Diaz-Sanchez and colleagues[68] also demonstrated nasal fluticasone muted increases in ragweed-specific IgE associated with combined challenge with diesel exhaust particles and ragweed pollen. Using an environmental exposure chamber, Ellis and colleagues[69] reported that diesel exhaust particles enhanced nasal response to ragweed allergen and that fexofenadine reduced pollutant-enhanced allergic rhinitis symptoms. Hernandez and colleagues[70] reported that pre-challenge dosing with anakinra inhibited airway inflammatory response to inhaled endotoxin (**Fig. 5**). Taken together, these observations provide proof of concept that antiinflammatory and allergy treatments may reduce inflammatory and allergic responses worsened by pollutants. However, these agents have not been tested for this purpose in randomized phase III clinical trials.

Nutraceutical interventions have also been examined as interventions for pollutant exposure. Romieu and colleagues[71] examined the effect of combination of vitamins C and E in children with asthma in a Mexican study. They observed that ozone reduced decreases in FEF 25% to 75% in children with homozygous for the GSTM1 null gene and that this antioxidant prophylaxis reduced the effect of ozone on lung

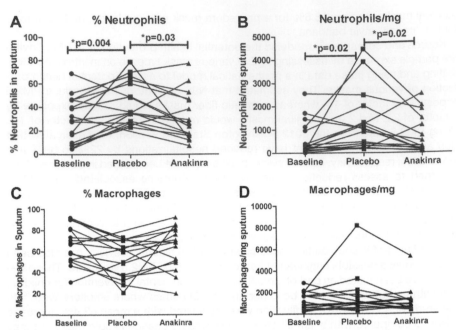

Fig. 5. Anakinra pretreatment reduces airway neutrophilia after LPS exposure. Percentage neutrophils (*A*), neutrophils per milligram of sputum (*B*), percentage macrophages (*C*), and macrophages per milligram of sputum (*D*) were determined from induced sputum samples taken at the baseline visit and 4 hours after inhaled LPS challenge with anakinra or placebo treatment. Wilcoxon signed-rank tests were used to compare either post-LPS anakinra or placebo levels with baseline levels. A linear mixed-model approach was used to calculate the treatment effect comparing anakinra with placebo. (*From* Hernandez ML, Mills K, Almond M, et al. IL-1 receptor antagonist reduces endotoxin-induced airway inflammation in healthy volunteers. *J Allergy Clin Immunol.* Feb 2015;135(2):379-85. https://doi.org/10.1016/j.jaci.2014.07.039.)

function. In a controlled exposure study with ozone, Chen and colleagues[72,73] observed that fish oil that is rich in omega-3 polyunsaturated fatty acids reduced ozone-induced decreases in lung function. In 2 studies, Hernandez and colleagues[74] and Burbank and colleagues[75] determined that pretreatment with gamma tocopherol, an isoform of vitamin E, reduced endotoxin-induced airway neutrophilia. Sulforaphane, which is an inducer of NRF2-regulated antioxidant enzymes, has been reported to reduce inflammatory response to diesel exhaust particle challenge.[76] However, sulforaphane treatment did not prevent ozone-induced inflammation in a proof-of-concept study.[77] Taken together, these studies suggest a potential role for nutraceutical prophylaxis to prevent pollutant-induced exacerbation. However, as with pharmacologic interventions, these approaches have not been studied in large phase III clinical trials for this purpose. Furthermore, in some cases, there may be only specific subgroups, such as GSTM1 null individuals with vitamin C and E intervention, who may benefit from these approaches.

Policy Interventions

Although personal interventions deserve more study, policy-based interventions are the most effective approach to reduce airborne pollutants and improve human health.

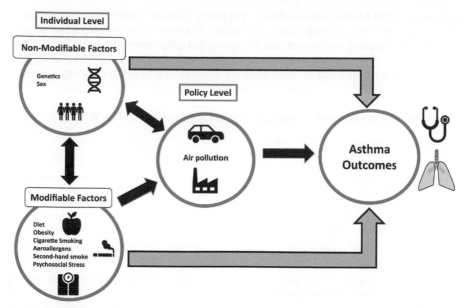

Fig. 6. Modifiable and non-modifiable factors should be considered when developing policies to mitigate air pollution health effects.[83]

There are examples of policy interventions that have been shown to reduce pollutant-induced adverse health effects. In 1996, Atlanta implemented changes in automobile traffic patterns as a condition of hosting the Olympic Games.[78] With these changes, there was a reduction in ozone levels and in asthma events as reflected in the Georgia Medicaid claims file. Short-term policy changes involving alternate-day driving privileges were effective in reducing PM2.5 pollution during the 2008 Beijing Olympics.[79] Longer term policy changes have also been shown to reduce air pollution with improved health outcomes. Reduced air pollution in Southern California across several years due to statewide air quality policies has been associated with improved lung growth in children and reduced acute episodes of lung disease due to pollution.[80,81] Specifically, reduced PM2.5, but not PM10 or ozone, was associated with reduced asthma incidence.[82]

SUMMARY

Anticipated changes in the distribution and concentration of ambient air pollutants influenced by climate and weather are projected to magnify the future scope and health impacts of respiratory and related allergic disorders if ignored. Several factors affect susceptibility to air pollutant–induced disease, as reviewed by Stevens and colleagues.[83] Potentially addressable factors that enhance risk for pollutant-induced disease include obesity, diets lacking in antioxidants, failure to avoid pollutant exposure, and increased psychosocial stress (to be reviewed by Dr Wright in another chapter of this issue). Social policy regarding housing quality and locating polluting industries near low-income housing is also addressable. Low-income housing, likely due to location near pollutant sources, is associated with greater pollutant exposure and worse asthma outcomes.[84] Using personal protective technology (masks and air filters) may be useful in reducing risk for pollutant-induced disease. Reducing BMI, consuming antioxidant-rich foods, reducing indoor pollutant sources (tobacco smoke, biomass fuels for heating and cooking), and better baseline control of asthma should also reduce risk for pollutant-induced disease. Pharmacologic interventions specifically for air pollutant exposures are intriguing but only tested in small laboratory-based studies. More important long-term measures will be policy interventions that promote or reward less use of fossil fuels for industry, transport, and energy generation as well as better land use and greenspace policies. Physicians can play a critical role in this by providing science-based health effects information to policymakers as they consider such policies. These approaches are depicted in **Fig. 6**.

CLINICS CARE POINTS

- Be aware of times of peak pollutant exposure by monitoring daily pollutant warnings offered by news outlets. Also, be aware that ozone levels are generated daily from reactions of ultraviolet light with volatile organic compounds and NOx, with peak levels occurring in the late afternoon. Use this information to avoid exposure to pollutants.
- Maintain good asthma control by use of antiinflammatory medication in conjunction with your health care provider.
- Consider use of masks or air filters to reduce exposure to PM2.5, especially if an acute pollution event (eg, wildfire) is occurring in your region.
- Be active as an advocate for clean air policies in your area.

FUNDING

Supported by Environmental Protection Agency Cooperative Agreement CR 84033801.

DISCLOSURE

The authors have nothing to disclose.

REFERENCES

1. Hernandez ML, Peden DB. Air pollution: indoor and outdoor. In: Burks AW, Holgate ST, O'Hehir RE, et al, editors. Middleton's allergy principles and practice. 9th edition. Philadelphia, PA: Elsevier; 2020. p. 479–99, chap 30.
2. Bernstein JA, Alexis N, Barnes C, et al. Health effects of air pollution. J Allergy Clin Immunol 2004;114(5):1116–23.
3. Burbank AJ, Peden DB. Assessing the impact of air pollution on childhood asthma morbidity: how, when, and what to do. Curr Opin Allergy Clin Immunol 2018;18(2):124–31.
4. Thurston GD, Balmes JR, Garcia E, et al. Outdoor Air Pollution and New-Onset Airway Disease. An Official American Thoracic Society Workshop Report. Ann Am Thorac Soc 2020;17(4):387–98.
5. Landrigan PJ, Fuller R, Acosta NJR, et al. The Lancet Commission on pollution and health. Lancet 2018;391(10119):462–512.
6. Pacheco SE, Guidos-Fogelbach G, Annesi-Maesano I, et al. Climate change and global issues in allergy and immunology. J Allergy Clin Immunol 2021;148(6): 1366–77.
7. Shea KM, Truckner RT, Weber RW, et al. Climate change and allergic disease. J Allergy Clin Immunol 2008;122(3):443–53.

8. Ziska LH. Climate, Carbon Dioxide, and Plant-Based Aero-Allergens: A Deeper Botanical Perspective. Front Allergy 2021;2:714724.
9. Anderegg WRL, Abatzoglou JT, Anderegg LDL, et al. Anthropogenic climate change is worsening North American pollen seasons. Proceedings of the National Academy of Sciences of the United States of America 2021;118(7). https://doi.org/10.1073/pnas.2013284118.
10. Ziska LH, Makra L, Harry SK, et al. Temperature-related changes in airborne allergenic pollen abundance and seasonality across the northern hemisphere: a retrospective data analysis. Lancet Planet Health 2019;3(3):e124–31.
11. Ziska L, Knowlton K, Rogers C, et al. Recent warming by latitude associated with increased length of ragweed pollen season in central North America. Proceedings of the National Academy of Sciences of the United States of America 2011;108(10):4248–51.
12. Rauer D, Gilles S, Wimmer M, et al. Ragweed plants grown under elevated CO(2) levels produce pollen which elicit stronger allergic lung inflammation. Allergy 2021;76(6):1718–30.
13. Zhu C, Farah J, Choël M, et al. Uptake of ozone and modification of lipids in Betula Pendula pollen. Environ Pollut 2018;242(Pt A):880–6.
14. Rorie A. Climate Change Factors and the Aerobiology Effect. Immunol Allergy Clin North Am 2022;42(4):771–86.
15. Mendy A, Salo PM, Cohn RD, et al. House Dust Endotoxin Association with Chronic Bronchitis and Emphysema. Environ Health Perspect 2018;126(3):037007.
16. Mendy A, Wilkerson J, Salo PM, et al. Synergistic Association of House Endotoxin Exposure and Ambient Air Pollution with Asthma Outcomes. Am J Respir Crit Care Med 2019. https://doi.org/10.1164/rccm.201809-1733OC.
17. Thorne PS, Kulhankova K, Yin M, et al. Endotoxin exposure is a risk factor for asthma - The National Survey of Endotoxin in United States Housing. Am J Respir Crit Care Med 2005;172(11):1371–7. Not in File.
18. Mueller-Anneling L, Avol E, Peters JM, et al. Ambient endotoxin concentrations in PM10 from Southern California. Environ Health Perspect 2004;112(5):583–8.
19. Carty CL, Gehring U, Cyrys J, et al. Seasonal variability of endotoxin in ambient fine particulate matter. J Environ Monit 2003;5(6):953–8. Not in File.
20. Gent JF, Triche EW, Holford TR, et al. Association of low-level ozone and fine particles with respiratory symptoms in children with asthma. JAMA 2003;290(14):1859–67.
21. Wei Y, Qiu X, Sabath MB, et al. Air Pollutants and Asthma Hospitalization in the Medicaid Population. Am J Respir Crit Care Med 2022;205(9):1075–83.
22. Bi J, D'Souza RR, Moss S, et al. Acute Effects of Ambient Air Pollution on Asthma Emergency Department Visits in Ten U.S. States. Environ Health Perspect 2023;131(4):47003.
23. Altman MC, Kattan M, O'Connor GT, et al. Associations between outdoor air pollutants and non-viral asthma exacerbations and airway inflammatory responses in children and adolescents living in urban areas in the USA: a retrospective secondary analysis. Lancet Planet Health 2023;7(1):e33–44.
24. Gehring U, Wijga AH, Hoek G, et al. Exposure to air pollution and development of asthma and rhinoconjunctivitis throughout childhood and adolescence: a population-based birth cohort study. Lancet Respir Med 2015;3(12):933–42.
25. Zhang Y, Wei J, Shi Y, et al. Early-life exposure to submicron particulate air pollution in relation to asthma development in Chinese preschool children. J Allergy Clin Immunol 2021;148(3):771–82.e12.

26. Hsu HH, Chiu YH, Coull BA, et al. Prenatal Particulate Air Pollution and Asthma Onset in Urban Children. Identifying Sensitive Windows and Sex Differences. Am J Respir Crit Care Med 2015;192(9):1052–9.

27. Bose S, Chiu YM, Hsu HL, et al. Prenatal Nitrate Exposure and Childhood Asthma. Influence of Maternal Prenatal Stress and Fetal Sex. Am J Respir Crit Care Med 2017;196(11):1396–403.

28. Diaz-Sanchez D, Dotson AR, Takenaka H, et al. Diesel exhaust particles induce local IgE production in vivo and alter the pattern of IgE messenger RNA isoforms. J Clin Invest 1994;94(4):1417–25.

29. Diaz-Sanchez D, Garcia MP, Wang M, et al. Nasal challenge with diesel exhaust particles can induce sensitization to a neoallergen in the human mucosa. J Allergy Clin Immunol 1999;104(6):1183–8.

30. Diaz-Sanchez D, Tsien A, Casillas A, et al. Enhanced nasal cytokine production in human beings after in vivo challenge with diesel exhaust particles. J Allergy Clin Immunol 1996;98(1):114–23.

31. Burbank AJ, Sood AK, Kesic MJ, et al. Environmental determinants of allergy and asthma in early life. J Allergy Clin Immunol 2017;140(1):1–12.

32. Scannell C, Chen L, Aris RM, et al. Greater ozone-induced inflammatory responses in subjects with asthma. Am J Respir Crit Care Med 1996;154(1):24–9. Not in File.

33. Hernandez ML, Lay JC, Harris B, et al. Atopic asthmatic subjects but not atopic subjects without asthma have enhanced inflammatory response to ozone. J Allergy Clin Immunol 2010;126(3):537–44.

34. Hernandez M, Brickey WJ, Alexis NE, et al. Airway cells from atopic asthmatic patients exposed to ozone display an enhanced innate immune gene profile. J Allergy Clin Immunol 2012;129(1):259–61.

35. Alexis NE, Zhou LY, Burbank AJ, et al. Development of a screening protocol to identify persons who are responsive to wood smoke particle-induced airway inflammation with pilot assessment of GSTM1 genotype and asthma status as response modifiers. Inhal Toxicol 2022;34(11–12):329–39.

36. Alexis NE, Huang YC, Rappold AG, et al. Patients with asthma demonstrate airway inflammation after exposure to concentrated ambient particulate matter. Am J Respir Crit Care Med 2014;190(2):235–7.

37. Hernandez ML, Herbst M, Lay JC, et al. Atopic asthmatic patients have reduced airway inflammatory cell recruitment after inhaled endotoxin challenge compared with healthy volunteers. J Allergy Clin Immunol 2012;130(4):869–876 e2.

38. Peden DB, Setzer RW Jr, Devlin RB. Ozone exposure has both a priming effect on allergen-induced responses and an intrinsic inflammatory action in the nasal airways of perennially allergic asthmatics. Am J Respir Crit Care Med 1995;151(5):1336–45.

39. Bascom R, Naclerio RM, Fitzgerald TK, et al. Effect of ozone inhalation on the response to nasal challenge with antigen of allergic subjects. Am Rev Respir Dis 1990;142(3):594–601.

40. Peden DB, Boehlecke B, Horstman D, et al. Prolonged acute exposure to 0.16 ppm ozone induces eosinophilic airway inflammation in asthmatic subjects with allergies. J Allergy Clin Immunol 1997;100(6 Pt 1):802–8.

41. Rusznak C, Devalia JL, Davies RJ. Airway response of asthmatic subjects to inhaled allergen after exposure to pollutants. Thorax 1996;51(11):1105–8.

42. Boehlecke B, Hazucha M, Alexis NE, et al. Low-dose airborne endotoxin exposure enhances bronchial responsiveness to inhaled allergen in atopic asthmatics. J Allergy Clin Immunol 2003;112(6):1241–3.

43. Chen LL, Tager IB, Peden DB, et al. Effect of ozone exposure on airway responses to inhaled allergen in asthmatic subjects. Chest 2004;125(6):2328–35.

44. Hanania NA, Tarlo SM, Silverman F, et al. Effect of exposure to low levels of ozone on the response to inhaled allergen in allergic asthmatic patients. Chest 1998; 114(3):752–6.

45. Ball BA, Folinsbee LJ, Peden DB, et al. Allergen bronchoprovocation of patients with mild allergic asthma after ozone exposure. J Allergy Clin Immunol 1996; 98(3):563–72.

46. Kehrl HR, Peden DB, Ball B, et al. Increased specific airway reactivity of persons with mild allergic asthma after 7.6 hours of exposure to 0.16 ppm ozone. J Allergy Clin Immunol 1999;104(6):1198–204.

47. Ørby PV, Bønløkke JH, Bibby BM, et al. Dose-response curves for co-exposure inhalation challenges with ozone and pollen allergen. Eur Respir J 2019;54(2).

48. Eldridge MW, Peden DB. Allergen provocation augments endotoxin-induced nasal inflammation in subjects with atopic asthma. J Allergy Clin Immunol 2000;105(3):475–81.

49. Schaumann F, Muller M, Braun A, et al. Endotoxin augments myeloid dendritic cell influx into the airways in patients with allergic asthma. Am J Respir Crit Care Med 2008;177(12):1307–13.

50. Rider CF, Yamamoto M, Günther OP, et al. Controlled diesel exhaust and allergen coexposure modulates microRNA and gene expression in humans: Effects on inflammatory lung markers. J Allergy Clin Immunol 2016;138(6):1690–700.

51. Horne BD, Joy EA, Hofmann MG, et al. Short-Term Elevation of Fine Particulate Matter Air Pollution and Acute Lower Respiratory Infection. Am J Respir Crit Care Med 2018;198(6):759–66.

52. Lu W, Tian Q, Xu R, et al. Short-term exposure to ambient air pollution and pneumonia hospital admission among patients with COPD: a time-stratified case-crossover study. Respir Res 2022;23(1):71.

53. Bozack A, Pierre S, DeFelice N, et al. Long-Term Air Pollution Exposure and COVID-19 Mortality: A Patient-Level Analysis from New York City. Am J Respir Crit Care Med 2022;205(6):651–62.

54. Yee J, Cho YA, Yoo HJ, et al. Short-term exposure to air pollution and hospital admission for pneumonia: a systematic review and meta-analysis. Environ Health 2021;20(1):6.

55. Xu L, Taylor JE, Kaiser J. Short-term air pollution exposure and COVID-19 infection in the United States. Environ Pollut 2022;292(Pt B):118369.

56. Sheppard N, Carroll M, Gao C, et al. Particulate matter air pollution and COVID-19 infection, severity, and mortality: A systematic review and meta-analysis. Sci Total Environ 2023;880:163272.

57. Burbank AJ. Risk Factors for Respiratory Viral Infections: A Spotlight on Climate Change and Air Pollution. J Asthma Allergy 2023;16:183–94.

58. Monoson A, Schott E, Ard K, et al. Air pollution and respiratory infections: the past, present, and future. Toxicol Sci 2023;192(1):3–14.

59. Beentjes D, Shears RK, French N, et al. Mechanistic Insights into the Impact of Air Pollution on Pneumococcal Pathogenesis and Transmission. Am J Respir Crit Care Med 2022;206(9):1070–80.

60. Clapp PW, Sickbert-Bennett EE, Samet JM, et al. Evaluation of Cloth Masks and Modified Procedure Masks as Personal Protective Equipment for the Public During the COVID-19 Pandemic. JAMA Intern Med 2021;181(4):463–9.

61. Kodros JK, O'Dell K, Samet JM, et al. Quantifying the Health Benefits of Face Masks and Respirators to Mitigate Exposure to Severe Air Pollution. Geohealth 2021;5(9). e2021GH000482.
62. Morgan WJ, Crain EF, Gruchalla RS, et al. Results of a home-based environmental intervention among urban children with asthma. N Engl J Med 2004; 351(11):1068–80.
63. Cui X, Li Z, Teng Y, et al. Association Between Bedroom Particulate Matter Filtration and Changes in Airway Pathophysiology in Children With Asthma. JAMA Pediatr 2020;174(6):533–42.
64. Allen RW, Barn P. Individual- and Household-Level Interventions to Reduce Air Pollution Exposures and Health Risks: a Review of the Recent Literature. Curr Environ Health Rep 2020;7(4):424–40.
65. Vagaggini B, Taccola M, Conti I, et al. Budesonide reduces neutrophilic but not functional airway response to ozone in mild asthmatics. Am J Respir Crit Care Med 2001;164(12):2172–6.
66. Holz O, Tal-Singer R, Kanniess F, et al. Validation of the human ozone challenge model as a tool for assessing anti-inflammatory drugs in early development. J Clin Pharmaco 2005;45(5):498–503.
67. Alexis NE, Lay JC, Haczku A, et al. Fluticasone propionate protects against ozone-induced airway inflammation and modified immune cell activation markers in healthy volunteers. Environ Health Perspect 2008;116(6):799–805.
68. Diaz-Sanchez D, Tsien A, Fleming J, et al. Effect of topical fluticasone propionate on the mucosal allergic response induced by ragweed allergen and diesel exhaust particle challenge. Clin Immunol 1999;90(3):313–22.
69. Ellis AK, Murrieta-Aguttes M, Furey S, et al. Effect of fexofenadine hydrochloride on allergic rhinitis aggravated by air pollutants. ERJ Open Res 2021;7(2). https://doi.org/10.1183/23120541.00806-2020.
70. Hernandez ML, Mills K, Almond M, et al. IL-1 receptor antagonist reduces endotoxin-induced airway inflammation in healthy volunteers. J Allergy Clin Immunol 2015;135(2):379–85.
71. Romieu I, Sienra-Monge JJ, Ramirez-Aguilar M, et al. Antioxidant Supplementation and Lung Functions among Children with Asthma Exposed to High Levels of Air Pollutants. Am J Respir Crit Care Med 2002;166(5):703–9.
72. Romieu I, Meneses F, Ramirez M, et al. Antioxidant supplementation and respiratory functions among workers exposed to high levels of ozone. Am J Respir Crit Care Med 1998;158(1):226–32.
73. Chen H, Tong H, Shen W, et al. Fish oil blunts lung function decrements induced by acute exposure to ozone in young healthy adults: A randomized trial. Environ Int 2022;167:107407.
74. Hernandez ML, Wagner JG, Kala A, et al. Vitamin E, gamma-tocopherol, reduces airway neutrophil recruitment after inhaled endotoxin challenge in rats and in healthy volunteers. Free Radic Biol Med 2013;60:56–62.
75. Burbank AJ, Duran CG, Pan Y, et al. Gamma tocopherol-enriched supplement reduces sputum eosinophilia and endotoxin-induced sputum neutrophilia in volunteers with asthma. J Allergy Clin Immunol 2018;141(4):1231–1238 e1.
76. Heber D, Li Z, Garcia-Lloret M, et al. Sulforaphane-rich broccoli sprout extract attenuates nasal allergic response to diesel exhaust particles. Food Funct 2014; 5(1):35–41.
77. Duran CG, Burbank AJ, Mills KH, et al. A proof-of-concept clinical study examining the NRF2 activator sulforaphane against neutrophilic airway inflammation. Respir Res 2016;17(1):89.

78. Friedman MS, Powell KE, Hutwagner L, et al. Impact of changes in transportation and commuting behaviors during the 1996 Summer Olympic Games in Atlanta on air quality and childhood asthma. JAMA 2001;285(7):897–905.
79. Liu Y, He K, Li S, et al. A statistical model to evaluate the effectiveness of PM2.5 emissions control during the Beijing 2008 Olympic Games. Environ Int 2012;44:100–5.
80. Gauderman WJ, Urman R, Avol E, et al. Association of improved air quality with lung development in children. N Engl J Med 2015;372(10):905–13.
81. Berhane K, Chang CC, McConnell R, et al. Association of Changes in Air Quality With Bronchitic Symptoms in Children in California, 1993-2012. JAMA 2016;315(14):1491–501.
82. Garcia E, Berhane KT, Islam T, et al. Association of Changes in Air Quality With Incident Asthma in Children in California, 1993-2014. JAMA 2019;321(19):1906–15.
83. Stevens EL, Rosser F, Forno E, et al. Can the effects of outdoor air pollution on asthma be mitigated? J Allergy Clin Immunol 2019. https://doi.org/10.1016/j.jaci.2019.04.011.
84. Schuyler AJ, Wenzel SE. Historical Redlining Impacts Contemporary Environmental and Asthma-related Outcomes in Black Adults. Am J Respir Crit Care Med 2022;206(7):824–37.

Extreme Weather Events and Asthma

Jennilee Luedders, MD*, Jill A. Poole, MD, Andrew C. Rorie, MD

KEYWORDS

- Asthma • Extreme weather • Thunderstorm asthma • Wildfires • Tropical cyclones
- Freshwater flooding • Temperature extremes • Climate change

KEY POINTS

- With climate change and global warming concerns, it can be anticipated that the world will continue to experience increased amounts of outdoor air pollution, increased pollen exposure and increased frequencies of extreme weather events.
- Thunderstorms, wildfires, tropical cyclones, freshwater flooding, and extreme temperatures can have devastating impacts on the respiratory health of affected populations, particularly those with asthma.
- Extreme weather events and their health effects disproportionately affect disadvantaged and lower socioeconomic populations.

INTRODUCTION

Asthmatics make up a population that is particularly vulnerable to serious health impacts from severe and extreme weather events such as thunderstorms, tornadoes, wildfires, droughts, floods, tropical storms, and extremes of temperature, among others. These weather events can drastically affect human health by causing injury, illness, death, as well as through socioeconomic influences.[1] Previous research has found positive associations with extreme heat/cold events, droughts, wildfires, and floods with negative influences on human health.[2] With persistent effects from climate change, it is anticipated we will continue to see increased frequency of extreme climate and weather events that have significant influences on allergic airway diseases such as asthma.[3]

Different environmental and social factors have varying degrees of influence on individuals affected by weather and climate changes and those with chronic health conditions, such as asthma, being particularly sensitive.[1] Extreme weather changes are capable of affecting airway hyperresponsiveness both directly, such as cold air, or indirectly by increasing aeroallergen levels and worsening air pollution.[4,5] Knowledge

Division of Allergy & Immunology, Department of Internal Medicine, University of Nebraska Medical Center, 985990 Nebraska Medical Center, Omaha, NE 68198, USA
* Corresponding author. 985990 Nebraska Medical Center, Omaha, NE 68198-5990.
E-mail address: jennilee.luedders@unmc.edu

Immunol Allergy Clin N Am 44 (2024) 35–44
https://doi.org/10.1016/j.iac.2023.07.001
0889-8561/24/© 2023 Elsevier Inc. All rights reserved.

of these weather events is critical for the allergy and immunology community to adequately address the influences of affected patient populations. In this article, we aim to review recent literature focused specifically on extreme weather events and associated health impacts on asthma. It is essential to increase awareness of these events so identification of potential medical needs of affected populations and improved planning for consequences of these extreme weather events.

THUNDERSTORM ASTHMA

One the most notable but rare extreme weather events with significant influences on asthma is known as "thunderstorm asthma." Thunderstorm asthma is a phenomenon where increased frequencies of asthma attacks are observed in geographic areas recently affected by thunderstorm events. These events have been observed in Australia, Saudi Arabia, North America, Iran, United Kingdom, Italy, Kuwait, and China.[6] The exact mechanism is not fully understood, and although various theories exist, one leading model is accepted as most likely. Namely, the presumed mechanism is excess pollen grains are released in the hours preceding a thunderstorm and undergo rupture due to osmotic swelling or electrostatic charge driven rupture with subsequent release of subpollen particles.[7] These small pollen fragments are then thought to be carried down to ground level within rain droplets or via cold downdrafts/outflows from thunderstorms.[8] Although typically large grass pollen would have settled in the upper airways, when ruptured into smaller fragments (<3 μm) they are able penetrate deeper into bronchial systems, leading to bronchospasm and asthma exacerbations.[6,7,9]

There are various molecular pathways suspected to be involved in thunderstorm asthma. In previous in vitro and ex vivo studies, it has been shown that allergens, including grass pollen, can prompt secretion of interleukin (IL)-8 from respiratory cells and thus lead to neutrophil recruitment to the airways, worsening asthma.[10–12] Additionally, other studies have suggested IL-4 as a potentiator of eosinophilic lung inflammation involved in thunderstorm asthma because IL-4 causes antibody isotype switching to IgE leading to allergic sensitization.[13,14]

To more closely examine weather parameters of thunderstorm-associated emergency department (ED) visits for asthma in the United States, Park and colleagues conducted a study analyzing more than 63,000 asthma-related ED visits in Louisiana.[15] The authors reported that on days where a thunderstorm occurred, for each 1 g/m^2/s higher daily precipitation rate, the risk of asthma-related ER visits was increased by 14.5% (relative rate [RR] 1.145 per 1 g/m^2/s [95% confidence interval (CI), 1.009–1.300]).[15] They also found that on thunderstorm days, for each 1°C lower daily mean temperature, there was an increased risk of asthma-related ER visits by 1.1% (RR = 1.011 per 1°C change [95% CI, 1.000–1.021]).[15] They specifically noted these risks to be higher among children and adults aged younger than 65 years.[15] In summary, this study suggested that higher amounts of rainfall and lower temperatures on thunderstorm days may contribute to more asthma attacks and weather forecast data may be helpful in predicting high-risk days for thunderstorm asthma.[15]

Both grass pollen and fungal spores are thought to be implicated in thunderstorm asthma.[6,16] Specifically, ryegrass (Lolium perenne) pollen sensitization has been suspected as a risk factor for thunderstorm asthma. The 2 main allergens in ryegrass pollen are Lol p 1 and Lol p 5, and each elicits serum IgE positivity in more than 90% of ryegrass pollen-sensitive patients.[17] Hew and colleagues investigated whether ryegrass pollen sensitization had diagnostic utility for predicting risk of thunderstorm asthma.[9] Specifically, they assessed serum-specific IgE levels for ryegrass pollen and for Lol p 1 and Lol p 5 specifically in 60 patients who presented to the ED for asthma during the 2016 Melbourne thunderstorm asthma event.[9] For comparison, they took samples from 19 control individuals with seasonal allergic rhinitis and were outdoors in Melbourne during the thunderstorm but did not develop thunderstorm asthma.[9] They found that patients with thunderstorm asthma had mean Lol p 1 IgE (1.28 μg/mL) levels similar to the control group (1.15 μg/mL) but increased mean levels of ryegrass pollen IgE (51.5 kU/L) and Lol p 5 IgE levels (2.61 μg/mL) versus controls (16.7 kU/L and 1.7 μg/mL, respectively).[9] Based on this data, they suggested that susceptibility to thunderstorm asthma was associated with higher levels of ryegrass pollen (and specifically Lol p 5) IgE sensitization.[9] The authors concluded that ryegrass pollen IgE levels might be a possible indicator for thunderstorm asthma risk and could potentially be used in the development of risk-prediction tools.[9]

In addition to pollen and fungi, biogenic volatile organic compounds (BVOCs) have been hypothesized to potentially play a role in thunderstorm asthma. In 2019, Gibbs and colleagues investigated the role of plant-related BVOCs on asthma with the hypothesis that increased BVOC emissions may contribute to thunderstorm asthma.[18] They took 14 volunteers with seasonal asthma and recorded respiratory symptoms, peak expiratory flow levels, and collected BVOC concentrations from ambient air from a suburban backyard of a privately owned home.[18] They found substantially increased levels of BVOCs including linalool (honey fragranced terpene), hexenal (aldehyde sensitizer), and hexanoic acid before a thunderstorm.[18] They also demonstrated that increased levels of linalool predicted increased asthma symptoms including wheeze and dry cough.[18] The authors concluded that BVOCs may play a role in contributing to thunderstorm asthma, although further studies are warranted.[18]

In another study, Elliot and colleagues performed an analysis of routinely collected health-care data in England and focused on June of 2021 where significant increases in health-care utilization were noted immediately following a period of thunderstorm activity.[19] On June 16, 2021, there were several localized thunderstorms categorized as weak to moderate storms that occurred across England.[19] They analyzed population health impacts on the following day and found that there was a notable spike in asthma symptoms in the areas affected by these storms.[19] Specifically, ED visits for asthma increased by 560% compared with the expected average from the previous 4 weeks.[19] Primary care out-of-hours contacts increased by 349% and ambulance calls increased by 54%.[19] Those aged between 5 and 44 years were the age group most affected.[19]

Interestingly, these respiratory health impacts in England linked to thunderstorm activity were not as clear as previous episodes because several of the storms that led to increased asthma symptoms were defined as "weak" rather than "severe" storms.[19] The explanation for this observation was suggested to be driven by strikingly increased levels of grass pollen demonstrated during these storm events.[19] It was postulated that meteorologic conditions (humidity, convergent crosswinds, and gust fronts) associated with storms were driving events versus specific lightning activity.[19] Thus, future studies should expand definitions to include not only thunder/lightning storms but also "storm" or "severe weather" events to understand the phenomenon of thunderstorm asthma.[19]

Along these lines, to examine whether increased pollen levels alone or lightning presence alone may be associated with severe asthma, Smith and colleagues investigated thunderstorm asthma events in Minnesota from 2007 to 2018.[20] They looked at the risk of severe asthma events at any time thunderstorm asthma conditions occurred, not only during the most severe storms or during highest pollen levels.[20] On the days of thunderstorms (defined as 2 or more lightning strikes) with high pollen counts (>75th percentile) of any type (tree, grass weed), there was a higher risk of asthma-related ED visits (RR = 1.047, CI 1.012–1.083) when compared with days without a thunderstorm asthma event.[20] In contrast, exposure to lightning strikes in the presence of low-pollen levels (<25th percentile) or exposure to high pollen levels without the presence of lightning strikes did not demonstrate association with increased severe asthma-related ED visits.[20] The authors concluded that these results were consistent with the hypothesis that thunderstorm asthma is a unique environmental and health phenomenon associated with co-occurrence of both thunderstorm activity and high pollen levels.[20]

One of the critical lessons learned from these thunderstorm asthma events is that a significant portion of affected individuals are those without previously known airway disease (potentially up to 60%).[6,21] Because seasonal allergic rhinitis and higher ryegrass pollen-specific IgE concentrations are thought to be risk factors for thunderstorm asthma,[6,21] allergists are in a unique position to potentially identify patients without a history of asthma who may be at risk for future adverse consequences related to a thunderstorm asthma event. Educating patients on behavioral interventions such as avoiding outdoor exposure in the hours around thunderstorms and monitoring grass pollen counts[21] particularly in regards to the seasonal timing of thunderstorm asthma (April through June in United States/Europe/Canada, and October through December in Australia) may help with awareness.[22] Additionally, allergy immunotherapy and inhibition-specific allergic mediators could be considered as potential prevention strategies for thunderstorm asthma, particularly in those sensitive to grass pollens.[6] Finally, emphasizing the importance of adherence to inhaled corticosteroids before and during a thunderstorm event can also help at-risk individuals already on these treatments.[6]

WILDFIRES

Climate change has increased drought conditions that are favorable for the development of wildfires and may result in serious health consequences.[23] Wildfires generate large amounts of air pollution including greenhouse gases, photochemically reactive compounds, and particulate matter.[24] We continue to learn more about the health impacts from wildfire smoke exposure but long-term health consequences from such exposures are largely unknown. It is critical to develop an understanding of the health impacts from wildfire smoke exposure on vulnerable populations to effectively mitigate these impacts.[25]

A study done by Heaney and colleagues investigated the association between wildfire smoke fine particular matter ($PM_{2.5}$) and cardiorespiratory-related hospital visits during wildfires that occurred between 2004 and 2009 in California.[26] They estimated daily mean wildfire-specific fine particulate matter using the Global Fire Emissions Database and defined "smoke event days" as days when the cumulative wildfire-specific $PM_{2.5}$ concentration was 98th percentile or greater.[26] It was demonstrated that smoke event days were associated with a 3.3% increase in hospital visits for all respiratory diseases (95% CI, 0.4%–6.3%).[26] When focused on asthma, smoke event days were associated with a 10.3% increase in hospital visits for asthma (95% CI, 2.3%–19.0%).[26] They also found that young children aged 0 to 5 years were most affected by these health effects.[26] They concluded that wildfire smoke exposure leads to substantially increased adverse health outcomes in affected populations and more aggressive prevention strategies are warranted.[26] Thus, improved evacuation plans, proper protective equipment, and statewide guidelines are necessary for future event planning.[26]

In addition, Beyene and colleagues examined prolonged wildfire smoke exposure in adults with severe asthma during an intense wildfire period in Australia from 2019 to 2020.[27] Participants who had been previously enrolled in an asthma registry completed a questionnaire including asthma symptoms and wildfire exposure.[27] They found that 83% of the participants had experienced respiratory symptoms including breathlessness, wheeze, and cough during the wildfire period and 44% required oral corticosteroid treatment of an asthma exacerbation during the wildfire.[27] Following the wildfire, 65% of the participants reported continued asthma symptoms but they also noted that treatment of asthma with various monoclonal antibody therapies (eg, mepolizumab, omalizumab, or benralizumab) was associated with a reduced risk of persistent symptoms (absolute risk reduction [aRR] 0.77, CI 0.60–0.99, $P = .046$).[27] It was concluded that wildfire exposure is associated with both acute and persistent respiratory symptoms in asthmatics.[27]

To determine whether respiratory health impacts due to particulate matter from wildfires differed from health impacts of particulate matter originating from other sources such as transportation or industry, Kiser and colleagues examined frequency of asthma exacerbations in EDs and urgent care centers in Reno, Nevada from 2013 to 2018 in relationship to wildfire smoke and particulate matter levels.[25] The presence of wildfire smoke increased the association of a 5 $\mu g/m^3$ increase in daily and 3-day averages of $PM_{2.5}$ with asthma visits by 6.1% and 6.8%, respectively.[25] For PM_{10}, the 5 $\mu g/m^3$ increase in daily and 3-day averages of PM_{10} associated asthma visits was increased by wildfire smoke presence by 5.5% and 7.2%, respectively.[25] In summary, there were stronger associations of $PM_{2.5}$ and PM_{10} with asthma emergent/urgent care visits when wildfire smoke was present when compared with nonwildfire PM suggesting that wildfire-related PM may be more harmful for asthmatics than PM from other sources.[25]

TROPICAL CYCLONES

Due to effects of climate change and global warming, there has been an increased frequency and severity of floods and cyclones.[28] Model projections predict that global tropical cyclone precipitation rates will increase by 14% with a 2°C increase in mean temperature.[29] Previous studies have suggested that hurricane exposure has led to increases in self-reported asthma attacks following the hurricane events, as demonstrated by studies of Hurricane Katrina where prevalence of an asthma exacerbation prehurricane and posthurricane were 4.4% and 9.1%, respectively ($P < .0001$).[30] Additionally, increased moisture associated with storms and flooding leads to increased humidity and dampness in the built environment, which supports growth of both molds and dust mites, allergens recognized to exacerbate asthma symptoms.[23]

Ramesh and colleagues investigated changes in ED visits associated with floods due to Tropical Storm Imelda that occurred in 2019 in southeastern Texas.[31] They found that during the flood period, ED visits due to asthma had increased by 10% (95% CI: 1%–19%) in the flooded areas when compared with nonflooded areas of Texas.[31] Another study by Lee and colleagues examined the effects of Hurricane Maria in Puerto Rico in 2017, on the development of respiratory disease in children in infants that were in utero exposed and conceived at least 5 months after the hurricane.[32] They examined the nasal microbiome of all the infants and found that infants in the Hurricane Maria exposure group were more likely to have a *Staphylococcus-Streptococcus* dominant microbiome when compared with the control group of infants without exposure to Hurricane Maria.[32] This finding suggests that infants may be at increased risk of asthma because earlier studies have reported that infants with

Staphylococcus or *Streptococcus*-dominant nasal microbiomes have higher risks of asthma.[32,33]

FRESHWATER FLOODING

Asthma exacerbations have been linked with flooding events in several previous studies.[5,34,35] Although most of these earlier studies link asthma with hurricane-associated flooding events, freshwater flooding may also be associated with asthma due to long-term exposure to mold, fungi, and endotoxins.[36] In 2021, Larson and colleagues conducted surveys of households in Detroit, Michigan, whereby recurrent home flooding secondary to storm-water events occurred.[36] They demonstrated that having at least one adult with asthma living in the home was positively associated with a history of flooding (OR 1.42, 95% CI 1.22–1.64).[36] Moreover, renters and communities of color were disproportionally affected by flooding events.[36]

Another study investigating the effects of freshwater flooding was conducted by Kontowicz and colleagues in 2022 and focused on the state of Iowa.[37] Iowa experiences flooding about 20 days of the year, exposing many residents to the negative health effects from flooding,[37] such as dampness and mold presence, increasing the odds of respiratory infections.[38] This study aimed to determine the associations between areas with flooding and influenza diagnoses.[37] In many hosts, influenza leads to only mild infection, whereas those with chronic lung disease such as asthma, influenza can lead to serious risks such as hospitalization or death. Using de-identified influenza tests from a large private insurance database and the Iowa State Hygienic Laboratory, and established flooding frequency using stream height data from stream gauges, the authors reported a consistent 1% associated increase in influenza diagnoses per day of flooding (95% CI, 1.00–1.04).[37] The greatest risks were seen in the most densely populated areas of Iowa.[37] The authors postulated that if there were to be a widespread flooding event in the state (as seen in 2010), there could be an additional 31,555 influenza diagnoses in Iowa for each day of flooding.[37] Therefore, it was suggested that populations exposed to flooded areas consider taking measures to avoid environmental exposures in order to reduce possible health consequences from influenza.[37]

EXTREMES OF TEMPERATURE

Nonoptimum ambient temperature (more simply known as low and high temperatures) is a known risk factor for premature death and there is growing evidence that it may also play a role in exacerbating asthma. Unfortunately, there are limited studies and the effects of temperature on asthma are inconsistently described.[39,40] A recent study conducted in China where nearly 5000 adult asthmatics were tracked from 2017 to 2020 and associations between daily pulmonary function tests and ambient temperature were assessed.[39] They found that when temperatures were elevated, there was a statistically significant decrease in forced expiratory volume in one second (FEV_1) by 26 mL (95% CI: 4.9–47, $P < .05$).[39] The effects on lung function of the extreme high temperatures were noted to occur at around 24 hours after the peak temperature and could persist until 72 hours after the peak.[39] In contrast, the effects from extreme low temperatures were noted to onset at time 0 hours and could also last until 72 hours postexposure.[39] Extreme low temperatures were associated with statistically significant decreases in FEV_1 of 60.4 mL (95% CI, 38.1–82.7, $P < .05$) and 101.5 mL in forced vital capacity (95% CI, 66.3–136.6, $P < .05$).[39] These data suggest that both ends of temperature extremes can have adverse health influences for asthmatics but the effects of low temperature may be more deleterious.[39]

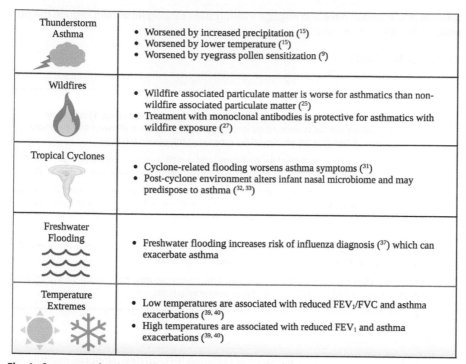

Thunderstorm Asthma	• Worsened by increased precipitation ([15]) • Worsened by lower temperature ([15]) • Worsened by ryegrass pollen sensitization ([9])
Wildfires	• Wildfire associated particulate matter is worse for asthmatics than non-wildfire associated particulate matter ([25]) • Treatment with monoclonal antibodies is protective for asthmatics with wildfire exposure ([27])
Tropical Cyclones	• Cyclone-related flooding worsens asthma symptoms ([31]) • Post-cyclone environment alters infant nasal microbiome and may predispose to asthma ([32, 33])
Freshwater Flooding	• Freshwater flooding increases risk of influenza diagnosis ([37]) which can exacerbate asthma
Temperature Extremes	• Low temperatures are associated with reduced FEV_1/FVC and asthma exacerbations ([39, 40]) • High temperatures are associated with reduced FEV_1 and asthma exacerbations ([39, 40])

Fig. 1. Summary of asthma effects associated with severe weather events. Asthma symptoms can be affected by various weather events including thunderstorms, wildfires, tropical cyclones, freshwater flooding, and temperature extremes. (Figure created with BioRender. com.)

A systematic meta-analysis (37 articles) review was conducted by Han and colleagues in 2022 to further assess the influences of extreme heat and cold on asthma.[40] Results demonstrated that the relative risk for an asthma exacerbation in extreme heat was 1.07 (95% CI, 1.03–1.12) and in extreme cold was 1.20 (95% CI, 1.12–1.29).[40] Therefore, this study further supports the role of extreme heat and extreme cold in negatively affecting respiratory health consequences in asthma, with greater potential risks with extreme cold conditions. However, in a literature review focused on the effects of ambient extreme heat and morbidity outcomes of pediatric populations, Uibel and colleagues in 2022 highlighted 4 studies from 2016 to 2019 demonstrating positive associations between asthma/wheeze morbidity and high temperature exposures.[41]

SUMMARY

With climate change and global warming concerns, it can be anticipated that the world will continue to experience increased amounts of outdoor air pollution, increased pollen exposure, and increased frequencies of extreme weather events.[23] A summary of asthma effects are highlighted in **Fig. 1**. These events can have devastating impacts on the respiratory health of affected populations, particularly those with asthma. Additionally, extreme weather events and their health effects disproportionately affect disadvantaged and lower socioeconomic populations.[23] The allergy and immunology community must be aware of the negative health effects of climate change-associated extreme weather events in order to adequately educate patients about health risks and engage in mitigation strategies to help reduce the potential adverse consequences.

CLINICS CARE POINTS

- Thunderstorm asthma is a phenomenon where increased frequencies of asthma exacerbations are seen in areas recently affected by thunderstorm events. This type of asthma exacerbation can be worsened by increased precipitation and lower temperature during the event. It can also be worsened by ryegrass pollen sensitization.
- Wildfires generate large amounts of air pollution and wildfire-associated particulate matter has been found to exacerbate asthma more than non–wildfire-associated particulate matter.
- Tropical cyclones can lead to subsequent flooding events, which contribute humidity and dampness and worsen asthma symptoms. Additionally, the postcyclone environment has been found to lead to alterations in infant nasal microbiomes and may predispose to asthma development later in life.
- Freshwater flooding can lead to an increased risk of influenza diagnosis and therefore could contribute to viral infections that lead to asthma exacerbations.
- Temperature extremes, such as both high and low temperatures, have been found to be associated with a reduction in FEV_1 and asthma exacerbations.

FUNDING AND DISCLOSURES

J.A. Poole has funding from Department of Defense (PR200793), National Institute for Occupational Safety and Health (U54OH010162 and R01OH012045), and Central States Center of Agricultural Safety and Health (CS-CASH). J.A. Poole has received research funding (reagent) from AstraZeneca and clinical site investigator from Takeda and GlaskoSmithKline.

REFERENCES

1. Bell JE, Brown CL, Conlon K, et al. Changes in extreme events and the potential impacts on human health. J Air Waste Manag Assoc 2018;68(4):265–87.
2. Weilnhammer V, Schmid J, Mittermeier I, et al. Extreme weather events in europe and their health consequences - A systematic review. Int J Hyg Environ Health 2021;233:113688.
3. Rorie A. Climate Change Factors and the Aerobiology Effect. Immunol Allergy Clin North Am 2022;42(4):771–86.
4. Poole JA, Barnes CS, Demain JG, et al. Impact of weather and climate change with indoor and outdoor air quality in asthma: A Work Group Report of the AAAAI Environmental Exposure and Respiratory Health Committee. J Allergy Clin Immunol 2019;143(5):1702–10.
5. Rorie A, Poole JA. The Role of Extreme Weather and Climate-Related Events on Asthma Outcomes. Immunol Allergy Clin North Am 2021;41(1):73–84.
6. Venkatesan P. Epidemic thunderstorm asthma. Lancet Respir Med 2022;10(4): 325–6.
7. Luschkova D, Traidl-Hoffmann C, Ludwig A. Climate change and allergies. Allergo J Int 2022;31(4):114–20.
8. Emmerson KM, Silver JD, Thatcher M, et al. Atmospheric modelling of grass pollen rupturing mechanisms for thunderstorm asthma prediction. PLoS One 2021; 16(4):e0249488.

9. Hew M, Lee J, Varese N, et al. Epidemic thunderstorm asthma susceptibility from sensitization to ryegrass (Lolium perenne) pollen and major allergen Lol p 5. Allergy 2020;75(9):2369–72.

10. Röschmann KI, Luiten S, Jonker MJ, et al. Timothy grass pollen extract-induced gene expression and signalling pathways in airway epithelial cells. Clin Exp Allergy 2011;41(6):830–41.

11. Röschmann K, Farhat K, König P, et al. Timothy grass pollen major allergen Phl p 1 activates respiratory epithelial cells by a non-protease mechanism. Clin Exp Allergy 2009;39(9):1358–69.

12. Blume C, Swindle EJ, Dennison P, et al. Barrier responses of human bronchial epithelial cells to grass pollen exposure. Eur Respir J 2013;42(1):87–97.

13. Massey O, Suphioglu C. Recent Advances in the Inhibition of the IL-4 Cytokine Pathway for the Treatment of Allergen-Induced Asthma. Int J Mol Sci 2021; 22(24). https://doi.org/10.3390/ijms222413655.

14. Busse WW. Biological treatments for severe asthma: A major advance in asthma care. Allergol Int 2019;68(2):158–66.

15. Park JH, Lee E, Fechter-Leggett ED, et al. Associations of Emergency Department Visits for Asthma with Precipitation and Temperature on Thunderstorm Days: A Time-Series Analysis of Data from Louisiana, USA, 2010-2012. Environ Health Perspect 2022;130(8):87003.

16. Davies J, Erbas B, Simunovic M, et al. Literature review on thunderstorm asthma and its implications for public health advice, 2017.

17. Singh MB, Hough T, Theerakulpisut P, et al. Isolation of cDNA encoding a newly identified major allergenic protein of rye-grass pollen: intracellular targeting to the amyloplast. Proc Natl Acad Sci U S A 1991;88(4):1384–8.

18. Gibbs JE. Essential oils, asthma, thunderstorms, and plant gases: a prospective study of respiratory response to ambient biogenic volatile organic compounds (BVOCs). J Asthma Allergy 2019;12:169–82.

19. Elliot AJ, Bennett CD, Hughes HE, et al. Spike in Asthma Healthcare Presentations in Eastern England during June 2021: A Retrospective Observational Study Using Syndromic Surveillance Data. Int J Environ Res Public Health 2021;18(23). https://doi.org/10.3390/ijerph182312353.

20. Smith ML, MacLehose RF, Chandler JW, et al. Thunderstorms, Pollen, and Severe Asthma in a Midwestern, USA, Urban Environment, 2007-2018. Epidemiology 2022;33(5):624–32.

21. Chatelier J, Chan S, Tan JA, et al. Managing Exacerbations in Thunderstorm Asthma: Current Insights. J Inflamm Res 2021;14:4537–50.

22. D'Amato G, Tedeschini E, Frenguelli G, et al. Allergens as trigger factors for allergic respiratory diseases and severe asthma during thunderstorms in pollen season. Aerobiologia 2019/06/01 2019;35(2):379–82.

23. Pacheco SE, Guidos-Fogelbach G, Annesi-Maesano I, et al. Climate change and global issues in allergy and immunology. J Allergy Clin Immunol 2021;148(6): 1366–77.

24. Urbanski SH, Min Wei, Baker, et al. Chemical composition of wildland fire emissions, vol. 8. Amsterdam, The Netherlands: Elsevier; 2009. Developments in environmental science.

25. Kiser D, Metcalf WJ, Elhanan G, et al. Particulate matter and emergency visits for asthma: a time-series study of their association in the presence and absence of wildfire smoke in Reno, Nevada, 2013-2018. Environ Health 2020;19(1):92.

26. Heaney A, Stowell JD, Liu JC, et al. Impacts of Fine Particulate Matter From Wildfire Smoke on Respiratory and Cardiovascular Health in California. Geohealth 2022;6(6). e2021GH000578.

27. Beyene T, Harvey ES, Van Buskirk J, et al. 'Breathing Fire': Impact of Prolonged Bushfire Smoke Exposure in People with Severe Asthma. Int J Environ Res Public Health 2022;19(12). https://doi.org/10.3390/ijerph19127419.

28. Takaro TK, Knowlton K, Balmes JR. Climate change and respiratory health: current evidence and knowledge gaps. Expert Rev Respir Med 2013;7(4):349–61.

29. Knutson T, Camargo SJ, Chan JCL, et al. Tropical Cyclones and Climate Change Assessment: Part II: Projected Response to Anthropogenic Warming. Bull Am Meteorol Soc 2020;101(3):E303–22.

30. Rath B, Young EA, Harris A, et al. Adverse respiratory symptoms and environmental exposures among children and adolescents following Hurricane Katrina. Public Health Rep 2011;126(6):853–60.

31. Ramesh B, Jagger MA, Zaitchik BF, et al. Estimating changes in emergency department visits associated with floods caused by Tropical Storm Imelda using satellite observations and syndromic surveillance. Health Place 2022;74:102757.

32. Lee S, Zhang A, Flores MA, et al. Prenatal exposure to Hurricane Maria is associated with an altered infant nasal microbiome. J Allergy Clin Immunol Glob 2022; 1(3):128–37.

33. Biesbroek G, Tsivtsivadze E, Sanders EA, et al. Early respiratory microbiota composition determines bacterial succession patterns and respiratory health in children. Am J Respir Crit Care Med 2014;190(11):1283–92.

34. Hayes D Jr, Jhaveri MA, Mannino DM, et al. The effect of mold sensitization and humidity upon allergic asthma. Clin Respir J 2013;7(2):135–44.

35. Tischer C, Chen CM, Heinrich J. Association between domestic mould and mould components, and asthma and allergy in children: a systematic review. Eur Respir J 2011;38(4):812–24.

36. Larson PS, Gronlund C, Thompson L, et al. Recurrent Home Flooding in Detroit, MI 2012-2020: Results of a Household Survey. Int J Environ Res Public Health 2021;18(14). https://doi.org/10.3390/ijerph18147659.

37. Kontowicz E, Brown G, Torner J, et al. Days of Flooding Associated with Increased Risk of Influenza. J Environ Public Health 2022;2022. 8777594.

38. Fisk WJ, Eliseeva EA, Mendell MJ. Association of residential dampness and mold with respiratory tract infections and bronchitis: a meta-analysis. Environ Health 2010;9:72.

39. Lei J, Peng L, Yang T, et al. Non-optimum ambient temperature may decrease pulmonary function: A longitudinal study with intensively repeated measurements among asthmatic adult patients in 25 Chinese cities. Environ Int 2022;164: 107283.

40. Han A, Deng S, Yu J, et al. Asthma triggered by extreme temperatures: From epidemiological evidence to biological plausibility. Environ Res 2023;216(Pt 2): 114489.

41. Uibel D, Sharma R, Piontkowski D, et al. Association of ambient extreme heat with pediatric morbidity: a scoping review. Int J Biometeorol 2022;66(8):1683–98.

The Impact of Climate Change on the Sporulation of Atmospheric Fungi

Young-Jin Choi, MD, PhD[a,b], Jae-Won Oh, MD, PhD[a,b],*

KEYWORDS

- Air pollution • Aeroallergens • Climate change • Pollen • Fungi • Pollutants • Allergy
- Fungal sensitization

KEY POINTS

- Climate change is projected to have potentially serious adverse consequences for human health.
- Allergenic and immune responses to a variety of environmental factors, such as pollens, fungi, and pollutants have been clearly demonstrated to be associated with an increased burden of upper and lower respiratory disease.
- Drought had a stronger effect on fungal community composition and induced greater functional loss. The magnitude of the fungal community change was directly proportional to the precipitation gradient.
- Recognition of climate-related environmental changes and their conseqent impact on respiratory allergy is paramount, as is working to lessen the impact on patients and adapting practices to meet those needs.

INTRODUCTION

The U.S. Global Change Research Program, Fourth National Climate Assessment reports that it is extremely likely that human activities, especially emissions of greenhouse gases, are the dominant cause of the observed warming since the mid-20th century. There are no convincing alternative explanations supported by observational evidence.[1] Asthma is a significant health and economic burden to patients, their families, and society, with 1.8 million emergency visits and 188,000 hospitalizations annually.[2] Though many factors have contributed to the increase in the prevalence of atopic diseases including asthma, observed changes in environmental factors, many related to the changing climate, are an important contributor. Coupled with

[a] Department of Pediatrics, College of Medicine, Hanyang University, Seoul, Korea;
[b] Department of Pediatrics, Hanyang University Guri Hospital, 153 Gyungchun-Ro, Guri, Gyunggi-Do 11923, Korea
* Corresponding author. Department of Pediatrics, Hanyang University Guri Hospital, 153 Gyungchun-Ro, Guri, Gyunggi-Do 11923, Korea.
E-mail address: jaewonoh@hanyang.ac.kr

Immunol Allergy Clin N Am 44 (2024) 45–54
https://doi.org/10.1016/j.iac.2023.07.005
0889-8561/24/© 2023 Elsevier Inc. All rights reserved.

increasing exposures to air pollution and other aeroallergens that have been linked to climate related changing trends in respiratory and allergic disease risk, climate effects on the distribution and concentration of fungi may also play a role.[3]

Atmospheric fungal spores have been linked with human respiratory allergies.[4,5] Atmospheric spore concentrations are influenced by a wide array of environmental, meteorologic, and biological factors and various interspecies interactions. Increase in atmospheric fungal spore concentrations have been associated with allergic rhinitis severity[6] and asthma hospital visits, admissions, and severity.[7,8] The number of spores in the atmosphere underlies seasonal variations, with climatic factors and circadian patterns influencing the spectrum of fungal species and their concentrations in the environment.[9,10] The number of spores in the air rises in particular in late summer and early autumn, while they diminish in winter. Considering daily fluctuations, the highest concentration of spore can be found in the afternoon and early evening.[10] However, knowledge on the determinants of spore production, seasonal dynamics, sources, and dispersion is still insufficient.[11,12]

A few spores of fungi are known to cause an allergic disease. *Alternaria alternata*, and *Cladosporium herbarium* can cause allergenic asthma and rhinitis.[10,13] *Cladosporium* spp. and *Alternaria* spp. spores are omnipresent in the environment and are two dominating genera in the total air spores. As *Alternaria* is a saprophyte living on most vegetation, the volumes of dust generated by combine harvesters will include many *Alternaria* spores which will be dispersed over a wide area. The threshold level of spore necessary to elicit allergic symptoms in sensitized patients is not known and varies between different species. Spore concentrations of *Alternaria* equal or greater than 100 spores/m^3 are believed to evoke allergic symptoms,[10,14] whereas the reference value for *Cladosporium* is estimated to be 3000 spores/m^3.[15]

THE CHANGE IN THE SPORULATION OF ATMOSPHERIC FUNGI

The influence of temperature and geographic location on seasonal indices of aerobiological particles has been confirmed in multiple studies. For example, the spatial pattern of *Alternaria* seasons has been shown to have a gradient of earlier start and longer duration from the south to the north of Europe.[16] Seasonal length, however, does not appear to correlate with *Alternaria* spore abundance: relatively short *Alternaria* seasons in northern locations can have higher seasonal spore integral (SSIn) values than those in locations with longer seasons.[16] A similar geographic pattern seems to be true for *Cladosporium*: longer seasons in the south with bimodal distributions and lower SSIn[6,17,18] than in central European locations with mono-modal *Cladosporium* distributions,[19–21] although *Cladosporium* incidence and seasonality are currently underreported.

There have been several reports demonstrating the long-term effect of climate change on pollen concentrations and seasonality.[22–26] In contrast to pollen, sources of airborne fungal spores are not straightforward. Fungal spore patterns are less clearly manifested with weaker rates of temporal changes than those for pollen.[27] However, grain crops and the process of harvesting were related to increase in both *Alternaria* and *Cladosporium* air concentrations.[28–31] Climate change has been reported to extend fungal fruiting seasons in Europe[32]; however, airborne *Cladosporium* and *Alternaria* conidia result from asexual reproduction, and thus the relationship between length of fruiting seasons and airborne spore abundance is not direct. The results of only few studies that have attempted to assess long-time trends in spore air concentrations are inconsistent, reporting increasing Alternaria and Cladosporium trends at one location, and decreasing at another, despite common increase in temperature.[16,21,33–35] Evaluating the impact of climate changes that have taken place during recent decades on airborne fungal spore concentrations and seasonality aids in modeling future exposures.

Changes in allergenic fungal species were evaluated and their concentration compared with the allergenic pollens in Seoul metropolitan, Korea (37°56′ N, 12°04′ E) for 25 years. Aerobiological monitoring of atmospheric fungal spores has been taking place in the Seoul metropolitan area of South Korea for 25 years (from January 1. 1998 to December 31. 2022), Burkard 7 days sampler was installed in Seoul metropolitan, South Korea and mold spores were collected, identified and counted every day. By using Weather data from National Weather Service, we investigated accumulated temperature, precipitation, and relative humidity, are the most influential variables to mold living. Aerobiological monitoring of atmospheric fungal spores has been taking place in the Seoul metropolitan, South Korea since 1998. This study focused on the evaluation of change of allergenic fungal species and their concentration for 25 years (submitted to Allergy Asthma Immunol Research (AAIR), **Fig. 1**).[36] There have been a few long-term detailed studies of concentration and seasonal variation of allergic fungi spores in the outdoors.[37,38]

It has become apparent that the spore concentration of *Alternaria* and *Cladosporium* have decreased and *Cladosporium* peak daily concentrations had a statistically significant annual decrease toward lower values for the last 25 years (submitted to AAIR, **Figs. 2** and **3**).[36] The trend of weather has changed to decreased precipitation in Seoul metropolitan, South Korea during the last 25 years (submitted to AAIR, **Fig. 4**).[36] It may suggest that the weather change such as atmospheric dryness and warming evaporated soils with silent droughts. Both *Cladosporium* and *Alternaria* daily spore concentrations exhibited little correlation with annual precipitation. This condition decreased the concentration of fungi, and even was not counted some certain fungi in Korea.

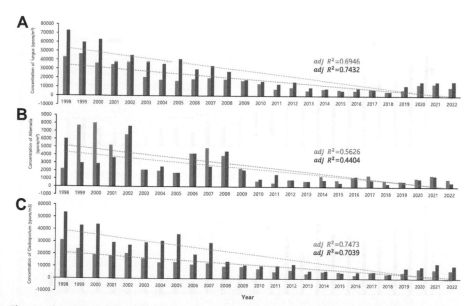

Fig. 1. Changes in the annual concentrations of the fungal spores in Seoul (*blue*) and Guri (*red*), Korea, for 25 years (1998–2022) (*A*) the concentration of total fungi. (*B*) the concentration of Alternaria, (*C*) the concentration of Cladosporium. (*With permission from* Allergy Asthma Immunol Research (AAIR). 2023 Nov;15(6)).

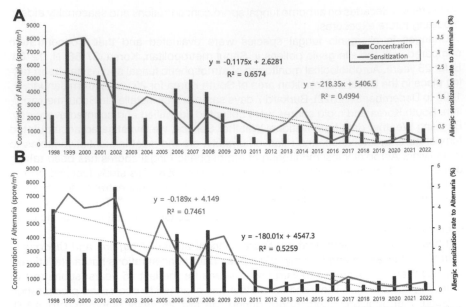

Fig. 2. Correlation between atmospheric concentration (*red bar*) and allergic sensitization rate (*blue line*) to Alternaria in (*A*) Seoul, (*B*) Guri. (*With permission from* Allergy Asthma Immunol Research (AAIR). 2023 Nov;15(6)).

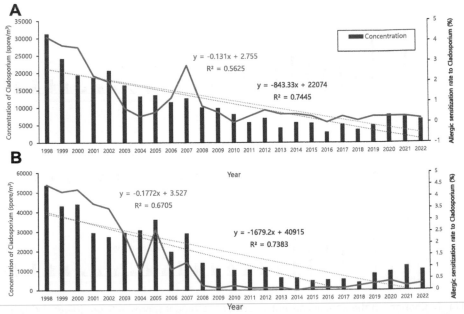

Fig. 3. Correlation between atmospheric concentration (*red bar*) and allergic sensitization rate (*blue line*) to Cladosporium in (*A*) Seoul, (*B*) Guri. (*With permission from* Allergy Asthma Immunol Research (AAIR). 2023 Nov;15(6)).

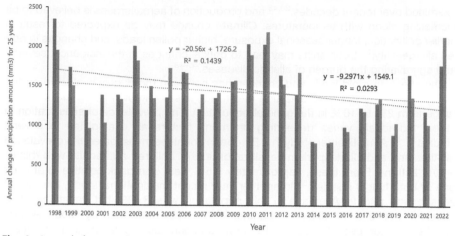

y = -20.56x + 1726.2
R² = 0.1439

y = -9.2971x + 1549.1
R² = 0.0293

Year

Fig. 4. Annual change of precipitation (mm3) in Seoul (*blue*) and Guri (*red*) for 25 years. (*With permission from* Allergy Asthma Immunol Research (AAIR). 2023 Nov;15(6)).

Climate change experts forecast widespsread changes in precipitation regimes, including longer, more intense droughts, causing desertification and promoting the expansion of drylands globally.[39] Drought had a stronger effect on fungal community composition and induced greater functional loss. The magnitude of the fungal community change was directly proportional to the precipitation gradient.[40] An experiment demonstrated how the exclusion of aerially dispersed fungi and bacteria altered the compositional and functional response of soil microbial and fungal communities to drought. The study presented that aerial dispersal rate alters soil microbial and fungal responses to disturbance. Changes in dispersal rates should be considered when predicting microbial and fungal responses to climate change.[41]

Long-term precipitation data are often available only at daily temporal resolution, that does not reflect high precipitation variability, and, therefore, cannot be used to relate spore concentrations to rainfall. Thus, in this study precipitation and RH had very weak negative correlation with Alternaria, and even weaker correlations with Cladosporium, such that precipitation was removed from the final stepwise regression model for Cladosporium. Likewise, daily cumulative precipitation was found to be the least important factor for *Alternaria* and *Cladosporium* spore concentrations in a recent study on long-term monitoring data (1987–2015) from 18 sites across Europe.[42]

It is known that *Cladosporium* and *Alternaria* spores whose concentration in the air is increased during hours with lower RH and higher temperatures. Average daily temperature is the main meteorologic factor affecting day-to-day variation in both genera.[43] However, observed annual changes in climate contradict the observed decline in *Alternaria* spore concentrations. Interestingly, in an experimental study with various temperatures, spores of *A alternata* were found to be decreasing along with the increase in temperatures, while mycelium growth was increasing, and the authors concluded that spore production in the future will be decreased.[44]

SENSITIZATION TO ALLERGIC FUNGI

Climate change is evident: rising temperatures are being observed and foreseen to increase worldwide. Multiple biological responses to changes in climate have been examined over recent decades,[20,45] and production of aeroallergens is believed to be increasing along with temperatures. Climate change may be expected to result in earlier pollination, longer seasonal exposure, higher pollen loads, and changes in pollen allergenicity.[22] Such shifts may lead to critical changes in the incidence, severity and aggravating the burden of allergic diseases.[46–48]

The effect on mold loads and changes has not been thoroughly evaluated on the allergic field. The exact sensitization rate to fungi is not known but is estimated to range from 2% to 10% in the general population. The prevalence of sensitization in atopic individuals varies depending on many factors as exemplified in several studies.[49–51] A multicenter study in 7 European countries investigated the prevalence of Alternaria and Cladosporium sensitization in 877 children and adults with rhinitis and/or asthma. From these, approximately 9.5% were skin prick positive to at least one or both fungal species.[52] In another very recent multinational study, the overall sensitization rate to Alternaria in this population was 3.7%, but variations were observed between the different countries.[53] A survey performed by Global Allergy and Asthma European Network in 16 European countries showed general sensitization rates of 11.9% for A alternata and 5.8% for Cladosporium herbarum with the highest prevalence in the UK, Ireland, and Northern Europe. The risk of asthma-related deaths is more than doubled when there is a high incidence of fungi spores and Alternaria is a known risk factor of asthma in childhood and young adulthood.[54,55]

Fungal communities play a major role as decomposers in the earth's ecosystems. Soils in terrestrial systems host biogeochemical transformations of important greenhouse gases. Soils might be drier with global warming increases evaporative water loss. The harmful impacts of acid rain on natural ecosystems include water contamination, soil acidification, and death to many organisms in last decades. The major sources of acid rain are sulfur dioxide and nitrogen oxides emitted into the atmosphere.[56]

SUMMARY

Coupled with air pollution and increases in exposure to aeroallergens, climate change is projected to have potentially serious adverse consequences for human health. Allergenic and immune responses to a variety of environmental factors, such as pollens, fungi, and pollutants have been clearly demonstrated to be associated with an increased burden of upper and lower respiratory disease.[2]

As reviewed herein, the sporulation of allergenic fungi is likely to be amplified as atmospheric CO_2 concentration increases with climate change, and is also likely to contribute to increasing prevalence and severity of asthma and the other respiratory allergies. Furthermore, global warming to drought and atmospheric dryness will continue to significantly alter the community composition and biochemical transformation of atmospheric allergic fungi.[26] Recognition of climate-related environmental changes and their conseqent impact on respiratory allergy is paramount, as is working to lessen the impact on patients and adapting practices to meet those needs.

CLINICS CARE POINTS

- Global warming to drought and atmospheric dryness will continue to significantly alter the community composition and biochemical transformation of atmospheric allergic fungi.
- Allergic sensitization rate to fungi will likely increase commensurate with increasing atmosphere allergenic fungi.

DISCLOSURE

Jae-Won Oh reports funding from the grant from Korean Academy of Pediatric Allergy and Respiratory Diseases (KAPARD, 1998-2007). This research was supported by the Research and Development grants for Weather, Climate, and Earth system Services of the National Institute of Meteorological Sciences, The Korea Meteorological Administration (2008-2018).); There were no relevant disclosures.

FUNDING

Funding from the grant from Korean Academy of Pediatric Allergy and Respiratory Diseases (KAPARD, 1998-2007). This research was supported by the Research and Development grants for Weather, Climate, and Earth system Services of the National Institute of Meteorological Sciences, The Korea Meteorological Administration (2008-2018).

REFERENCES

1. Crimmins A, Balbus JL, Gamble CB, et al, editors. The impacts of climate change on human health in the United States: a scientific assessment. Washington, DC: U.S. Global Change Research Program; 2016.
2. Sheehan WJ, Gaffin JM, Peden DB, et al. Advances in environmental and occupational disorders in 2016. J Allergy Clin Immunol 2017;140(6):1683–92.
3. Barnes CS, Alexis NE, Bernstein JA, et al. Reply. Journal of Allergy and Clinical Immunology: In Pract 2013;1(5):543–4.
4. Delfino RJ, Zeiger RS, Seltzer JM, et al. The effect of outdoor fungal spore concentrations on daily asthma severity. Environ Health Perspect 1997;105(6):622–35.
5. Barnes C. Fungi and Atopy. Clin Rev Allergy Immunol 2019;57(3):439–48.
6. Katotomichelakis M, Nikolaidis C, Makris M, et al. Alternaria and Cladosporium calendar of Western Thrace: Relationship with allergic rhinitis symptoms. Laryngoscope 2016;126(2):E51–6.
7. Atkinson RW, Strachan DP, Anderson I IR, et al. Temporal associations between daily counts of fungal spores and asthma exacerbations. Occup Environ Med 2006;63(9):580–90.
8. Stieb DM, Beveridge RC, Brook JR, et al. Air pollution, aeroallergens and cardiorespiratory emergency department visits in Saint John, Canada. J Expo Anal Environ Epidemiol 2000;10(5):461–77.
9. D'Amato G, Spieksma FT. Aerobiologic and clinical aspects of mould allergy in Europe. Allergy 1995;50(11):870–7.
10. Rodríguez-Rajo FJ, Iglesias I, Jato V. Variation assessment of airborne Alternaria and Cladosporium spores at different bioclimatical conditions. Mycol Res 2005; 109(Pt 4):497–507.
11. Kasprzyk I. Aeromycology–main research fields of interest during the last 25 years. Ann Agric Environ Med 2008;15(1):1–7.
12. Crameri R, Garbani M, Rhyner C, et al. Fungi: the neglected allergenic sources. Allergy 2014;69(2):176–85.
13. Caillaud D, Cheriaux M, Charpin D, et al. Outdoor moulds and respiratory health. Rev Mal Respir 2018;35(2):188–96.
14. Bernardis P, Agnoletto M, Puccinelli P, et al. Injective versus sublingual immunotherapy in Alternaria tenuis allergic patients. J Investig Allergol Clin Immunol 1996;6(1):55–62.

15. Darke CS, Knowelden J, Lacey J, et al. Respiratory disease of workers harvesting grain. Thorax 1976;31(3):294–302.
16. Skjøth CA, Damialis A, Belmonte J, et al. Alternaria spores in the air across Europe: Abundance, seasonality and relationships with climate, meteorology and local environment. Aerobiologia 2016;32(1):3–22.
17. Bardei F, Bouziane H, Trigo MDM, et al. Atmospheric concen- trations and intra-diurnal pattern of Alternaria and Cla- dosporium conidia in Tetouan (NW of Morocco). Aerobiologia 2017;33(2):221–8.
18. Almeida E, Caeiro E, Todo-Bom A, et al. The influence of meteorological param-eters on Alternaria and Cladosporium fungal spore concentrations in Beja (South-ern Portugal): Preliminary results. Aerobiologia 2018;34(2):219–26.
19. Chrenova J, Misik M, Scevkova J, et al. Monitoring of microscopic airborne fungi in Bratislava. Acta Fac Pharm Univ Comenianae 2004;51:68–72.
20. Kasprzyk I, Kaszewski BM, Weryszko-Chmielewska E, et al. Warm and dry weather accelerates and elongates Cladospo- rium spore seasons in Poland. Aerobiologia 2016;32(1):109–26.
21. Sindt C, Besancenot J-P, Thibaudon M. Airborne Cladosporium fungal spores and climate change in France. Aerobiologia 2016;32(1):53–68.
22. Lee KS, Kim KH, Choi YJ, et al. Increased sensitization rates to tree pollens in allergic children and adolescents and a change in the pollen season in the metro-politan area of Seoul, Korea. Pediatr Allergy Immunol 2021;32:872–9.
23. Park HJ, Lim HS, Park KH, et al. Changes in allergen sensitization over the last 30 years in Korea respira- tory allergic patients: a single-center. Allergy Asthma Im-munol Res 2014;6:434–43.
24. Kim JH, Oh JW, Lee HB, et al. Changes in sensitization rate to weed allergens in children with increased weeds pollen counts in Seoul metropolitan area. J Korean Med Sci 2012;27:350–5.
25. García-Mozo H, Yaezel L, Oteros J, et al. Statistical approach to the analysis of olive long-term pollen season trends in southern Spain. Sci Total Environ 2014; 473:103–9.
26. Bruffaerts N, De Smedt T, Delcloo A, et al. Comparative long-term trend analysis of daily weather conditions with daily pollen concentrations in Brussels, Belgium. Int J Biometeorol 2018;62(3):483–91.
27. Damialis A, Vokou D, Gioulekas D, et al. Long-term trends in airborne fungal-spore concentrations: a comparison with pollen. Fungal ecology 2015;13:150–6.
28. Friesen TL, De Wolf ED, Francl LJ. Source strength of wheat pathogens during combine harvest. Aerobiologia 2001;17(4):293–9.
29. Skjøth CA, Sommer J, Frederiksen L, et al. Crop harvest in Denmark and Central Europe contributes to the local load of airborne *Alternaria* spore concentrations in Copenhagen. Atmos Chem Phys 2012;12(22):11107–23.
30. Olsen Y, Begovic T, Skjøth CA, et al. Grain harvesting as a local source of Clado-sporium spp. in Denmark. Aerobiologia 2019;35.
31. Olsen Y, Gosewinkel UB, Skjøth CA, et al. Regional variation in airborne Alternaria spore concentrations in Denmark through 2012–2015 seasons: the influence of meteorology and grain harvesting. Aerobiologia 2019;35(3):533–51.
32. Boddy L, Büntgen U, Egli S, et al. Climate variation effects on fungal fruiting. Fungal Ecology 2014;10:20–33.
33. Corden JM, Millington WM. The long-term trends and seasonal variation of the aeroallergen Alternaria in Derby, UK. Aerobiologia 2001;17(2):127–36.

34. Corden JM, Millington WM, Mullins J. Long-term trends and regional variation in the aeroallergen Alternaria in Cardiff and Derby UK – are differences in climate and cereal production having an effect? Aerobiologia 2003;19(3):191–9.
35. Ščevková J, Dušička J, Mičieta K, et al. The effects of recent changes in air temperature on trends in airborne Alternaria, Epicoccum and Stemphylium spore seasons in Bratislava (Slovakia). Aerobiologia 2016;32(1):69–81.
36. Choi YJ, et al. Annual change of Fungal Sporulation and Allergic Sensitization Rate to Alternaria and Cladosporium in Korea over 25 years (1998 - 2022).
37. Grinn-Gofro'n A, Strzelczak A, Stèpalska D, et al. A 10-year study of Alternaria and Cladosporium in two Polish cities (Szczecin and Cracow) and relationship with the meteorological parameters. Aerobiologia 2016;32:83–94.
38. Anees-Hill S, Douglas P, Pashley CH, et al. A systematic review of outdoor airborne fungal spore seasonality across Europe and the implications for health. Sci Total Environ 2022;818:151716.
39. Schwalm CR, Anderegg WRL, Michalak AM, et al. Global patterns of drought recovery. Nature 2017;548(7666):202–5.
40. Ochoa-Hueso R, Collins SL, Delgado-Baquerizo M, et al. Drought consistently alters the composition of soil fungal and bacterial communities in grasslands from two continents. Global Change Biol 2018;24(7):2818–27.
41. Evans SE, Bell-Dereske LP, Dougherty KM, et al. Dispersal alters soil microbial community response to drought. Environ Microbiol 2020;22(3):905–16.
42. Grinn-Gofron' A, Mika A. Selected airborne aller- genic fungal spores and meteorological factors in Szczecin, Poland, 2004–2006. Aerobiologia 2008;24(2):89.
43. Aira M-J, Rodríguez-Rajo F-J, Fernández-Gonzalez M, et al. Cladosporium airborne spore incidence in the environmental quality of the Iberian Peninsula. Grana 2012;51(4):293–304.
44. Damialis A, Mohammad AB, Halley JM, et al. Fungi in a changing world: Growth rates will be elevated, but spore production may decrease in future cli- mates. Int J Biometeorol 2015;59(9):1157–67.
45. Walther GR. Community and ecosystem responses to recent climate change. Philos Trans R Soc Lond B Biol Sci 2010;365(1549):2019–24.
46. Cecchi L, D'Amato G, Ayres JG, et al. Projections of the effects of climate change on allergic asthma: the contribution of aerobiology. Allergy 2010;65(9):1073–81.
47. D'Amato G, Holgate ST, Pawankar R, et al. Meteorological conditions, climate change, new emerging factors, and asthma and related allergic disorders. A statement of the World Allergy Organization. World Allergy Organ J 2015;8(1):25.
48. M DA, Cecchi L, Annesi-Maesano I, et al. News on Climate Change, Air Pollution, and Allergic Triggers of Asthma. J Investig Allergol Clin Immunol 2018;28(2):91–7.
49. Bousquet J, Heinzerling L, Bachert C, et al. Practical guide to skin prick tests in allergy to aeroallergens. Allergy 2012;67(1):18–24.
50. Lyons TW, Wakefield DB, Cloutier MM. Mold and Alternaria skin test reactivity and asthma in children in Connecticut. Ann Allergy Asthma Immunol 2011;106(4):301–7.
51. Park HJ, Lee JH, Park KH, et al. A nationwide survey of inhalant allergens sensitization and levels of indoor major allergens in Korea. Allergy Asthma Immunol Res 2014;6(3):222–7.
52. D'Amato G, Chatzigeorgiou G, Corsico R, et al. Evaluation of the prevalence of skin prick test positivity to Alternaria and Cladosporium in patients with suspected respiratory allergy. A European multicenter study promoted by the Subcommittee on Aerobiology and Environmental Aspects of Inhalant Allergens of

the European Academy of Allergology and Clinical Immunology. Allergy 1997; 52(7):711–6.

53. de Benedictis FM, Franceschini F, Hill D, et al. The allergic sensitization in infants with atopic eczema from different countries. Allergy 2009;64(2):295–303.

54. Targonski PV, Persky VW, Kelleher P, et al. Characteristics of hospitalization for asthma among persons less than 35 years of age in Chicago. J Asthma 1995; 32(5):365–72.

55. Tariq SM, Matthews SM, Stevens M, et al. Sensitization to Alternaria and Cladosporium by the age of 4 years. Clin Exp Allergy 1996;26(7):794–8.

56. Dai Z, Liu X, Wu J, et al. Impacts of simulated acid rain on recalcitrance of two different soils. Environ Sci Pollut Res Int 2013;20(6):4216–24.

Impact of Climate Change on Indoor Air Quality

Alina Gherasim, MD[a], Alison G. Lee, MD, MS[b],
Jonathan A. Bernstein, MD[c],*

KEYWORDS

- Climate change • Indoor air quality • Pollutants • Allergy • Asthma

KEY POINTS

- Our climate has measurably changed over the years, which could be the greatest health threat of the twenty-first century.
- Climate change is affecting our ecosystems with consequent direct and indirect impact on our patients with allergic and respiratory diseases.
- Indoor air quality is a major concern worldwide due to its adverse effects on human health, which has the greatest impact on children and the elderly living in the lower socioeconomic strata of the population with allergic rhinitis, asthma, and chronic obstructive pulmonary disease.
- Lifestyle adjustments and implementation of effective evidence-based regulations can mitigate continued climate-related increases in indoor air pollution and consequently reduce the onset and progression of respiratory diseases.

BACKGROUND

Our climate has measurably changed over the years with globally averaged carbon dioxide (CO_2) concentration increasing from 250 to 410 ppm (www.ipcc.ch). Worldwide, the number of record cold days and nights has fallen, and the number of record hot days and nights has risen (www.ipcc.ch). Forecasts based on current data and computer modeling suggest that the Earth's surface temperature will continue to rise, oceans will continue to warm and absorb more CO_2, and sea levels will continue to rise. These natural system changes might be the greatest health threat of this century

[a] ALYATEC Environmental Exposure Chamber, 1 Place de l'Hôpital, Strasbourg, France; [b] Division of Pulmonary, Critical Care and Sleep Medicine, Icahn School of Medicine at Mount Sinai, 1 Gustave L Levy Place, New York, NY 10029, USA; [c] Division of Rheumatology, Allergy and Immunology, University of Cincinnati College of Medicine, 231 Albert Sabin Way, Cincinnati, OH 45267, USA
* Corresponding author. University of Cincinnati College of Medicine, Department of Internal Medicine, Division of Rheumatology, Allergy and Immunology, 231 Albert Sabin Way, ML#563, Cincinnati, Ohio 45267-0563.
E-mail address: bernstja@ucmail.uc.edu

Immunol Allergy Clin N Am 44 (2024) 55–73
https://doi.org/10.1016/j.iac.2023.09.001

as their adverse effects on both indoor and outdoor air quality are growing having the greatest impact on children and the elderly living in the lower socioeconomic strata of the population with allergic rhinitis (AR), asthma, and chronic obstructive pulmonary disease (COPD).[1–3]

Indoor air quality (IAQ) refers to the quality of the air in and around buildings and structures, with particular reference to the health and comfort of building occupants. IAQ has become a significant concern worldwide due to its increasingly documented adverse effects on immediate and long-term human health. Urban and economic growth has continued to rise over the past three decades, and consequently, energy consumption and CO_2 emissions from burning fossil fuels have led to increased air pollution.[4] The presence of aerosols and chemicals over the World Health Organization (WHO) allowable limits,[5] including chemical volatile organic compounds (cVOCs), particulate matter (PM) ranging from 0.1 to 10 µm, and aromatic hydrocarbons contributes to outdoor air pollution which becomes indoor air pollution when windows are open and there are inadequate measures to filter outdoor air coming indoors.[6,7]

According to the WHO, 7 million premature deaths are caused each year by the combined effects of ambient and household air pollution. Millions more are impacted by breathing polluted air. In 2019, 4.1 million deaths were caused by ambient air pollution alone, whereas household air pollution from cooking with polluting fuels caused approximately 2.3 million deaths over the same period.[8]

Epidemiologic studies indicate that climate change and indoor air pollution affect respiratory health, including the increase in the prevalence of allergic diseases and asthma.[9] In the most populated regions in the world, there is a huge burden of both outdoor and indoor pollutants and household pollutants, increasing the risk factors for allergic diseases.[10] This is strongly related to urbanization and a spectrum of environmental factors. A retrospective study conducted from 2011 to 2012 in China demonstrated that early allergic symptoms in childhood were mainly associated with indoor environmental exposures and that physician-diagnosed allergic diseases later in life were related to both ambient air pollution and indoor environmental exposures.[11]

This article explores several ways that current and predicted changes in climate influences IAQs impact on respiratory health and related disorders. The discussion will also focus on mitigating the impact of climate change on IAQ, which seems to be the greatest challenge we currently face.

AIR POLLUTION

According to the WHO definition, "air pollution is a complex mixture of liquid droplets, solid particles, and gases."[5] Air pollution emanates from a wide variety of sources, including domestic fuel combustion, industrial smokestacks, vehicle exhaust, power generation, agricultural practices, open burning of waste, and desert dust to name a few. Air pollutants measured include fine and course (PM2.5) and (PM10) PM, which are particles with aerodynamic diameters ranging from less than 2.5 and 10 µm, respectively, ultrafine particles less than 0.1 µm, ozone (O_3), nitrogen dioxide (NO_2), carbon monoxide (CO), and sulfur dioxide (SO_2). Fine particulates can penetrate through the lungs and cause cardiovascular and respiratory diseases such as stroke, lung cancer, asthma, respiratory infections, and COPD.[8] Recent data have shown an association between exposure to high levels of air pollution and developmental psychological problems including symptoms of attention-deficit hyperactivity disorder, anxiety, and depression[12] which may also influence respiratory disease as discussed in another section of this special issue.

INDOOR AIR POLLUTION AND POLLUTANTS SOURCES

Climate change can affect the indoor environment through heat and mass transfer between the indoors and outdoors[13] through two fundamental ways. First, a direct response to global warming itself, with extreme weather phenomena such as frequent or violent hurricanes, leads to an increase in IAQ problems. Second, IAQ may be impacted by indirect actions taken to reduce emissions of greenhouse gases that can lead to increased concentrations of indoor air contaminants. For example, large quantities of energy used for heating, cooling, dehumidifying, and humidifying are intentionally vented or accidently leaked from buildings. Reducing intentional ventilation rates or air-sealing an enclosure to reduce accidental infiltration not only reduces greenhouse gas emissions but also lowers a building's total ventilation rate. The main cause of IAQ problems are from sources that release gases or particles into the air with inadequate ventilation. Lower general ventilation rates increase the concentration of indoor contaminants such as CO_2, NO_2, and $O3$. High humidity levels and temperatures can also increase concentrations of certain pollutants.[14]

Carbon monoxide (CO) is an odorless, colorless gas released by fuel-burning stoves and heaters. A third of the world's population uses solid fuels derived from biomass or coal for cooking, heating, or lighting. These human activities, such as the burning of coal and oil often used in open fires or simple stoves with incomplete combustion, cause significant domestic air pollution when the smoke is poorly evacuated. Depending on the quantity breathed in, CO can have a negative impact on human health. The elderly, babies, pregnant women, and people suffering from heart and lung disease are even more sensitive to high levels of CO. Very high levels can be fatal. When CO is emitted into the atmosphere, it influences the quantity of greenhouse gases, which are linked to climate change and global warming. Consequent rising land and sea temperatures are altering ecosystems, increasing storm activity and causing other extreme weather phenomena[4] that in turn can impact respiratory health.

Ozone (O3) is an irritant gaseous pollutant with higher levels near the top of urban canyons compared with street-level concentrations.[15] Its impact on lung function, exacerbation of chronic respiratory diseases, increases in respiratory hospital admissions is well established.[16] Exposure to ozone increases the risk of sensitization to airborne allergens in predisposed individuals.[17] Infiltration from outdoors is the dominant factor affecting indoor ozone concentrations during heat waves.[18] Climate change not only effects the pollutants needed to create ground-level ozone but also influences chemical and physical processes that create ozone, and the transport of ozone, and its precursors.

Aromatic hydrocarbons such as polyaromatic hydrocarbons (PAHs) are persistent organic pollutants produced from industrial and domestic food processing.[19-21] Their sources are incomplete irritation, on of wood, oil, coal, gas, petrol gas and diesel, industrial electricity generation, and waste incineration that affect human health.[19] Acute exposures to high concentrations of these pollutants can cause inflammatory diseases.[22]

Inorganic air pollutants such as CO, CO_2, O3, NOx, and SO_2 have been demonstrated to induce asthma and bronchitis symptoms. Long-term exposure to these gases can cause chronic lung disease and loss of the senses of smell and taste.[23]

PM consists of airborne droplets and solid particles with different sizes, origins, and chemical compositions.[24] They are classified according to their aerodynamic diameter into four fractions: ultrafine (<0.01 μm), fine (0.01–2.5 μm), coarse (2.5–10 μm), and large (10–100 μm).[25] In the indoor environment, paints, varnishes, solvents, cleaning products, and office equipment such as photocopiers, printers, and gas stoves release PM.[26] If their airborne concentration is high, it will have a direct negative impact on the respiratory system. The upper respiratory tract is mainly affected by PM10, whereas the lower respiratory tract and alveoli are damaged by particles of size 2.5 μm and ultrafine particles of 0.1 μm or smaller.[27–29] Long-term exposure to airborne particles below the allowed limit has been shown to increase the risk of lung cancer,[24] asthma, bronchial irritation, and lung fibrosis.[8]

Indoor Allergens and Infections

The main sources of allergens in indoor environments are house dust mites, molds, pets, plants, and insects.[30,31] Specific immunoglobulin E (IgE) hypersensitivity is one of the main health problems caused by poor IAQ in damp homes.[32,33] Common indoor molds such as *Penicillium spp* and *Aspergillus spp* can induce IgE-mediated hypersensitivity, however, hypersensitivity pneumonitis, a type III-mediated immune response, can also occur when buildings are contaminated with bacteria and molds.[34] Allergic bronchopulmonary aspergillosis and allergic fungal sinusitis occur when these respiratory tracts colonized by molds elicit in situ allergic inflammatory reactions.[35,36] Most mold-related health issues pertain to microbial volatile organic compounds (mVOCs), which are the musty mildew odors that are smelled in mold-contaminated homes and buildings.

In modern homes, the warm and potentially humid indoor climate is ideal for the proliferation of dust mites and molds, increasing the risk of exposure to their allergenic proteins. Climate change can affect the ecosystem leading to altered patterns and levels of allergen exposures as well as earlier onset and longer exposure to seasonal aeroallergens. Infiltration of allergens into the indoor environment varies according to building's ventilation rate. Intense rainfall and flooding can cause dampness and mold proliferation in homes, which affects IAQ.[37–39] High levels of bacteria, mold, dust mites, animal dander, and pollen can be compounded due to inadequate housekeeping and humidity control, two controllable measures that can be taken to mitigate these exposures.

COVID-19 leading to increased indoor air pollutant exposure

The COVID-19 global pandemic has increased the time people spend indoors making them more vulnerable to indoor air pollutants. One study evaluated IAQ of 70 homes in the room where the worker performed telework activities (kitchens, bedrooms, offices, or living rooms) and repeated testing for 41 workers who returned to their higher educational institute workplace after mandatory teleworking at home ended. The levels of CO_2, CO, formaldehyde, PM (<10, 5, 2.5, 1, 0.5, and 0.3 μm and ultrafine) and levels of thermal comfort were measured at both sites.[40] Although most homes and higher educational institute sites had good IAQ, there were areas where concentrations of some pollutants were above legal standards, which was associated with increased symptoms in workers. These results demonstrate that the need to monitor air quality in the home and workplace of workers with prolonged indoor confinement as controlling ventilation, temperature, and humidity can reduce or prevent symptoms related to indoor air pollutants. Furthermore, improvement in various climatic parameters, such as temperature and humidity, can reduce or potentially prevent the emergence of new coronaviruses by modifying susceptibility factors in the host, the vectors, and the virus itself.[41]

Other sources of indoor air pollution are combustion and electrical appliances that emit O3, tobacco products, building materials furniture made from certain pressed wood products, floor coverings, and other furnishings that can emit chemical VOCs (cVOCs), household cleaning products that emit cVOCs, excess humidity that can promote mold, and dust mite growth can cause or aggravate chronic rhinitis and asthma.

Since the mid-1980s, the frequency and duration of the wildfire season has increased in the northwestern United States.[42] This phenomenon is linked to changes in forest management practices and climatological factors such as higher spring and summer temperatures, earlier snowmelt and moisture deficits. During exceptional events such as wildland fire, the infiltration of PM2.5 ambient wildland fire smoke into indoor environments is a determinant factor in increasing indoor air pollution levels.

Outdoor air pollution can enter a building through infiltration and both mechanical and natural ventilation. In the process known as infiltration, outdoor air enters buildings through openings, or cracks in walls, floors, and ceilings, as well as around doors and windows. Air movements associated with infiltration and natural ventilation are caused by differences in temperature between indoors and outdoors. When natural or mechanical ventilation is low, the air renewal rate is low and pollutant levels can increase. A conceptual diagram showing how indoor and outdoor air pollution including pollutant sources contribute to poor IAQ is shown in **Fig. 1**.

INDOOR AIR QUALITY STANDARDS

In Western countries, people spend around 90% of their time indoors,[43] where the concentrations of certain pollutants can often be higher than typical outdoor levels.[44]

IAQ guideline standards aimed to maintain healthy air in building are generated by several regulatory government and professional organizations including the Centers for Disease Control and Prevention,[45] the Occupational Safety and Health Administration, and the American Society of Heating, Refrigerating and Air-Conditioning Engineers.[46] The WHOs Air Quality Guidelines (AQGs) serve as global recommendations for national, regional, and city governments to improve the health of their citizens by reducing air pollution.[47] They integrate known scientific evidence of air pollution on health with monitoring each country's air quality progress. In 2021, the WHO revised the permissible limits for various air pollutants[4] (**Table 1**). Specifically, the annual mean value for PM10 was reduced to 15 $\mu g/m^3$ and for PM2.5 was reduced to 5 $\mu g/m^3$.

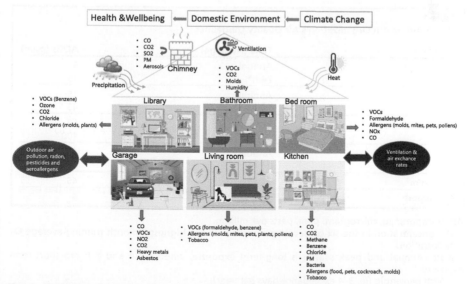

Fig. 1. Graphical abstract. Indoor air pollutants and sources.

Because office workers spend around 22 hours a day indoors and up to 40 hours a week in office buildings, in closed environments indoor air pollution can have a greater effect on health than outdoor air pollution. These effects can be mitigated by controlling indoor temperatures using well-maintained cooling systems that prevent the need to open windows and by adjusting airflow ventilation.[48,49] Vardoulakis and colleagues[50] identified location, building characteristics, and occupant behavior as the most important factors that influence indoor heat risks.

Location

Building location can have implications for indoor pollutants. Highways and busy areas are sources of particles and other pollutants in buildings. Buildings built on land with a high water table can cause water or chemical pollutants to seep into the building.[43] A study conducted in the United Kingdom has shown that high indoor temperatures cause more health issues in the bedroom (26°C) compared with living rooms or other living areas (28°C).[50] Monitoring campaigns show that temperatures are generally lower at night and early in the morning and rise gradually during the day peaking in the evening.[51,52]

Building Characteristics

Building design can also contribute to indoor air pollution. How energy is conserved through building practices can have an essential impact on occupants' respiratory health. In the past, buildings had high air exchange rates, ensuring that pollutants generated indoors were constantly diluted with outside air. However, unless outdoor climatic conditions are complementary to those desired indoors, these air changes require energy to condition the air to ensure health and comfort indoors. The natural ventilation reduction caused by outdoor air pollutants ranges from 40% to 70% in the most polluted area, whereas 5% to 20% in all other tested cities.[53] Poor-quality foundations, roofs, facades, and window and door openings can allow the intrusion of pollutants or water. Outside air intakes placed close to sources of pollutants

Table 1
The World Health Organization's Air Quality Guidelines

Pollutant	Time (Average)	AQGs (ppm)
PM2.5, $\mu g/m^3$	Annual	5
	24-h[a]	15
PM10, $\mu g/m^3$	Annual	15
	24-h[a]	45
O_3, $\mu g/m^3$	Peak season[b]	60
	8-h[a]	100
NO_2, $\mu g/m^3$	Annual	10
	24-h[a]	25
SO_2, $\mu g/m^3$	24-h[a]	40
CO, mg/m^3	24-h[a]	4

Abbreviations: μg, microgram; ppm, parts per million.
O_3 concentration in the six consecutive months with the highest 6-month running-average O_3 concentration.
Note: Annual and peak season is long-term exposure, whereas 24 and 8 h are short-term exposure.
[a] 99th percentile (ie, 3–4 exceedance days per year).
[b] Average of the daily maximum 8-h mean.

such as combustion products and waste containers are reintroduced into the indoor ambient air. In addition, multi-tenant buildings may require specific assessments to ensure that emissions from one unit do not permeate into another adjacent units.[54]

Occupant Behavior

Occupants' behavior depends on their age, and socioeconomic status.[54] Populations such as the elderly, isolated people, lower socioeconomic groups, as well as the very young, and people with preexisting health conditions are more vulnerable than others, to heat-related mortality and morbidity. This risk may reflect underlying medical conditions and physiologic vulnerability.[3] When the heating, ventilation, and air-conditioning (HVAC) system is not properly working, the building is often depressurized, and external pollutants can infiltrate the building. During painting and other renovations, dust and other building material by-products can be sources of pollutants circulating in the building.[44]

CONSEQUENCES OF INDOOR AIR POLLUTION ON ALLERGIC RHINITIS AND ASTHMA

AR and asthma have pathophysioologic links, known as the "united airways phenomenon,"[55] and represent the most common respiratory conditions.[56,57] Its increasing prevalence is strongly related to individual lifestyles.[58]

Indoor air pollution's impact on health is amplified by the amount of time spent indoors. Environmental factors such as NO_2, tobacco smoke, VOCs, and indoor allergens have all been associated with exacerbations of asthma and rhinitis.[59] PM10 may activate distinct inflammatory pathways, which might independently contribute to asthma pathogenesis. The respiratory epithelium of patients with severe asthma releases alarmin cytokines (eg, Thymic stromal lymphopoietin [TSLP], IL-25, IL-33) when exposed to PM compared with healthy subjects.[60]

Indoor allergens induce more severe allergic airway phenotypes than seasonal outdoor allergens. Sensitization to pet allergens is detected in 15% of the population, with a high degree of cross-reactivity between different species.[61] In cat owners' homes, up to 50% of airborne Fel d 1 is associated with particles greater than 10 μm in diameter, whereas around 23% of inhaled particles are smaller than 4.7 μm diameter. More than 50% of airborne Fel d 1 settles out between 30 minutes and 2 days of disturbance, but smaller particles can remain airborne for up to 14 days or longer.[62,63]

In contrast, 50% of asthmatics are sensitized to house dust mite (HDM).[61] In children with wheezing episodes, HDM sensitization is associated with greater bronchial inflammation and decreased lung function.[64]

CLIMATE CHANGE MITIGATION AND ADAPTATION MEASURES TO IMPROVE INDOOR AIR QUALITY

As buildings consume a substantial fraction of all energy carbon dioxide emissions to mitigate climate change, it is necessary to reduce the energy consumption of buildings. The benefit of thermal insulation of building envelopes improves thermal comfort and controls winter indoor temperatures. However, the negative impact includes the potential for increased risk moisture trapping, leading dampness and mold growth inside the walls that can permeate into the home over time. Energy efficiency measures in buildings are expected to be widely applied as climate change progresses.[65–67] Many energy efficiency measures in buildings will have a positive or negative influence on comfort conditions or IAQ. It is impossible to predict with any certainty the effect of energy efficiency in buildings given the impact of climate change may have on indoor environmental quality, comfort, and health.[68] According to extant literature, it is clear that comfort and health conditions can be improved through the strategic implementation of energy efficiency measures. Also, by reducing emissions from the combustion of fossil fuels, we can reduce air pollution and respiratory illnesses. These are just some of the many health benefits by implementing indoor pollution reduction measures.

Adaptation measures for flooding in the buildings consists on avoiding water entering the building by blocking all potential entry points, replacing carpets with vinyl or ceramic tiles, choosing building materials at risk for damage that can be easily replaced, using water-resistant paint, using furnishings with low VOC emissions, and more importantly maintaining optimal indoor ventilation.[51] Increased ventilation can reduce the permeability of the building envelope, thereby leading to the accumulation of indoor air pollutants such as particulates and environmental tobacco smoke.[69]

According to a recent review,[70] there is sufficient evidence that air filtration reduces indoor allergen levels. For households equipped with forced-air (HVAC) systems, regular maintenance programs along with use of high-efficiency disposable filters are important to maintain. Portable air purifiers equipped with new-generation high-efficiency particulate air filters seem to be beneficial in reducing cat allergen (Fel d 1) airborne concentration and reducing asthma exacerbations in allergic individuals.[71]

In some areas, new homes are required to have mechanical ventilation.[72] However, other studies reported problems related to installation and maintenance, which affect the reliability and performance of these systems.[73,74]

Diagnostic techniques used for IAQ evaluations are divided into a qualitative and a quantitative phase to measure relative humidity, room temperature, O_3, CO, CO_2, particulate concentrations, and microbial contaminants.[15] The primary worldwide studies[75–87] measuring indoor air pollutants levels and personal exposure inducing respiratory diseases are shown in **Table 2**.

The use of "green" construction materials in buildings may be seen as a climate change mitigation measure to reduce indoor pollution. Although this friendly environment may reduce pollutant emissions, the steel used has a negative impact by supporting microbial growth. Also, buildings can be constructed or adapted to be more flood-resistant by preventing floodwaters from entering a building, or by building construction interventions to minimize potential flood damage. Moreover, centrally installed ultraviolet irradiation units are methods that have been shown to be effective in reducing airway hyperresponsiveness and asthma symptoms in mold-sensitized asthmatic children with central home ventilation systems.[88]

Plants have the ability to absorb and catabolize toxic gases present in indoor and outdoor environments. Various plants, such as potted plants or green walls, are seen as potentially green solutions for improving IAQ and the health of inhabitants.[89] There are data demonstrating that indoor potted plants have the potential to reduce VOC concentrations in the indoor environment.[90]

Lifestyle adaptation can mitigate air pollution and climate change and indirectly reduce the onset and progression of respiratory diseases. Avoiding individual motorized transport is a simple and fundamental approach but not economically feasible until alternative forms of transportation such as electrical vehicles are accessible to all socioeconomic sectors of society. Outdoor exercise is also recommended, as its benefits should outweigh the negative effects of exposure to allergens and outdoor pollutants.[91] For pollen-allergic patients, it is recommended to limit time spent outdoors during high-pollen cycles and during high-traffic hours or warm days.[92] Air quality alerts, pollen calendars, and allergy diaries, among other mobile health tools can help plan outdoor activities, as well as control and monitor symptoms.[93]

Table 2
Main worldwide studies measuring indoor air pollutants levels and personal exposure inducing respiratory diseases

Author/Reference	Country	Participants	Indoor Pollution Assessments	Pollutant	Results
Cortez-Lugo et al,[74] 2008	USA	38 asthma children and COPD adults	MiniVol sampler, personal pumps, 2000	PM2.5 and PM10	Effects of PM exposure to lung function in asthma and COPD Decrease in MMEF in children with asthma with no medications
Cortez-Lugo et al,[75] 2015	Mexico	29 adults with COPD	Personal pumps, 2000	PM2.5	Reductions in peak expiratory flow and increased respiratory symptoms.
Cleary et al,[76] 2017	USA	2 cities	Formaldehyde Multimode Monitor, e P-Trak Ultrafine Particle Counter, E Q-Trak Indoor Air Quality Monitor,	VOCs, PM, CO	High CO concentrations with increased asthma symptoms
Delfino et al,[77] 2006	USA	48 asthmatic children	Personal PM2.5 monitor, Harvard impactor, 2003,2004.	PM2.5, NO2, elemental carbon	The positive association between FeNO and 2-d average pollutant concentrations. Strong associations were found for ambient elemental carbon and weak associations for ambient NO$_2$.

(continued on next page)

Table 2
(continued)

Author/Reference	Country	Participants	Indoor Pollution Assessments	Pollutant	Results
Fang et al,[78] 2019	China	20 asthma patients	Low-cost pump packages. 2017	VOCs	Associated health risks High levels of formaldehyde, acetaldehyde, and toluene in the bedrooms. Significant reductions in indoor VOCs with air cleaners
Jansen et al,[79] 2005	USA	16 asthma or COPD patients	Harvard Impactor, Marple Personal Environmental Monitors for PM10, 2002, 2003	PM2.5 and PM10	An increase in outdoor, indoor, and personal black carbon was associated with increases in FeNO but no significant association was found in spirometry, blood pressure, pulse rate, or SaO₂
Kearney et al,[80] 2011	Canada	Asthmatic children from 45 homes of nonsmoking adults and 49 homes of smoking adults	Portable condensation particle counter, 2005, 2006	UFP	A strong influence of cooking. Large indoor peaks and low infiltration of ambient PM resulted in the indoor sources contributing more than infiltrated UFP.
Rojas-Bracho et al,[81] 2000	USA	18 COPD patients	Modified PM2.5 and PM10 personal exposure monitor and a single personal pump, 1996, 1997	PM2.5, PM10	A strong association between PM2.5 indoor and outdoor levels and COPD

Author, Year	Country	Study	Method	Pollutants	Findings
Soppa et al,[82] 2014	Germany	55 healthy volunteers	Fast Mobility Particle Sizer, Aerodynamic Particle Sizer, Nanoparticle Surface Area Monitor	PM1, PM10, PM2.5	A strong association between high levels of indoor fine particles and decreases in lung function
Trenga et al,[83] 2006	USA	17 children, 57 elderly	Harvard Impactor, personal monitor, 1999–2001	PM2.5, PM10	MMEF was decreased in children with asthma without medications even though PM exposures were low for an urban area
Vardoulakis et al,[84] 2020		Systemic review		VOC, PM2.5, NO2	Cigarette smoking for PM2.5, gas appliances for NO2, and household products for VOCs, and PAHs are the main indoor pollutants. Home location near high-traffic-density roads, redecoration, and small house size contribute to high indoor air pollution. High indoor particulate matter, NO_2, and VOC levels were associated with respiratory symptoms, particularly asthma symptoms in children.
Weichenthal et al.[85] 2008		Review	Passive sampler	VOCs, UFP, NO2	A significant relationship between VOC exposure and asthma or related symptoms

(continued on next page)

Table 2
(continued)

Author/Reference	Country	Participants	Indoor Pollution Assessments	Pollutant	Results
Xia et al,[86] 2020	Hong Kong	20 COPD patients and 20 healthy participants	MicroPEM sensor, 2017–2018	PM2.5	Short-term exposure to PM2.5 results in an acute drop in SpO$_2$ in 0–3 h and insignificant at 0–12 h.

Abbreviations: CO, carbon monoxide; COPD, chronic obstructive pulmonary disease; FeNO, fraction of exhaled NO; MMEF, maximal mid-expiratory flow; NO$_2$, nitrogen dioxide; PM, particulate matter; UFP, ultra-fine particle; VOC, volatile organic compound.

DISCUSSION

Climate change can have several direct and indirect negative effects on the indoor environment that in turn impact respiratory health. These include overheating, indoor air pollution, biological contamination, flooding, and water damage. Climate change mitigation and adaptation measures in the residential construction sector involving improved building design and ventilation, passive cooling and energy efficiency measures can have beneficial effects on health, if properly designed and implemented. Even though there are many and varied methods for mitigating indoor pollution, we reviewed the most cited and efficient approaches. For example, the replacement of fossil fuels with renewable energy sources and the industry's commitment to a complete shift away from coal-fired power are necessary steps on the roadmap to a more environmentally friendly economy.[94] This approach will require a gradual transition depending on the availability of clean, affordable alternative forms of energy. The impact of air pollution on individuals' health will be devastating in the next decades if we do not curb projected trends.

Ventilation is an essential aspect of influencing IAQ, humidity-related allergens, and thermal comfort in homes. Behavioral aspects of building occupancy and energy-saving thermal efficiency improvements can compromise IAQ and increase indoor temperatures.[95] For this reason, the ventilation performance of energy-efficient homes requires further investigation.

The allergy and broader scientific community need to be aware of how atmospheric conditions influence increasing levels of air pollutants and aeroallergens, as well as their effects on health and how these exposures can be mitigated in the indoor environment. Adaptation practices must be implemented on an ongoing basis to meet the needs of vulnerable populations. Major technical advances have made buildings and vehicles more efficient and renewable energy sources much more cost-effective. Worldwide, financial resources are abundant, but are not allocated adequately to address modifiable factors that can affect climate change. Political commitment should ensure that policies focused on mitigating climate change should be implemented. Governments need to adopt effective, evidence-based regulations, as policy interventions are the only way to achieve significant improvements at the population level. All these efforts are crucial steps on the road to cleaner air and, ultimately, the prevention and reduction of respiratory diseases. These include investments in ecosystem processes that increase green spaces where marginalized vulnerable groups reside and by improving access to quality health care.

SUMMARY

The effects of weather and climate change on indoor and outdoor air quality are many and varied. Air pollution and climate change are closely linked, with air pollutants contributing to atmospheric temperature and rising temperatures due to climate change leading to an increase in natural VOCs emissions. In addition, CO_2 emissions mainly from fossil fuel combustion are not only a major driver of climate change but also major sources of air pollutants and increased tree and weed pollination.

Reducing the main risk factors for respiratory disease, particularly indoor and outdoor air pollution which as discussed are interrelated, is necessary to impact their burden on respiratory allergies. The exact consequences of these trends are uncertain, but the allergist community needs to be well informed in understanding the effects of air pollution on allergies and asthma, and the possible ways to mitigate their negative health consequences. The approach to climate change should be integrated and anticipatory to protect and treat patients with asthma and other allergic and climate-sensitive diseases from triggers that are likely driving this phenomenon. Climate and weather conditions will continue to change and could have a devastating effect on our planet. This issue has been heralded as the greatest global health threat of the twenty-first century.[96–98]

Overall, climate change is likely to act as a risk modifier in the indoor environment by potentially amplifying existing health risks. Well-targeted, cost-effective adaptation and mitigation measures could minimize these risks and provide associated health benefits.

DISCLOSURE

The authors have nothing to disclose.

REFERENCES

1. Poole JA, Barnes CS, Demain JG, et al. Impact of weather and climate change with indoor and outdoor air quality in asthma: A Work Group Report of the AAAAI Environmental Exposure and Respiratory Health Committee. J Allergy Clin Immunol 2019;143:1702–10.
2. Mertz O, Halsnæs K, Olesen JE, et al. Adaptation to Climate Change in Developing Countries. Environ Manag 2009;43:743–52.
3. Grecequet M, DeWaard J, Hellmann JJ, et al. Climate vulnerability and human migration in global perspective. Sustainability 2017;9:720.
4. U.S. Environmental Protection Agency (EPA). IPCC, W. "Working group I contribution to the IPCC fifth assessment report: climate change 2013: the physical science basis, summary for policymakers."IPCC, UN 2013. Available at: https://www.epa.gov/indoor-air-quality-iaq/introduction-indoor-air-quality. Accessed June 8, 2023.
5. World Health Organisation Report. 9 out of 10 people worldwide breathe polluted air, but more countries are taking action. Available at: http://www.who.lnt/news-room/detail/02-05-2018-9-out-of-10-people-worldwide-breathe-polluted-air-but-more-countries-are-taking-action. Accessed July 1, 2020.
6. Gawronski SW, Gawronska H, Lomnicki S, et al. Plants in air phytoremediation. In: Advances in botanical research, vol. 83. Amsterdam, Netherlands: Elsevier Ltd.; 2017. p. 319–46.
7. Wei X, Lyu S, Yu Y, et al. Phytoremediation of air pollutants: exploiting the potential of plant leaves, leaf-associated microbes. Front Plant Sci 2017;8:1–23.
8. World Health Organization. Top Ten Causes of Death. Available at: https://www.who.int/news-room/fact-sheets/detail/the-top-10-causes-of-death. Accessed February 25, 2022.
9. Deng SZ, Jalaludin BB, Antó JM, et al. Climate change, air pollution, and allergic respiratory diseases: a call to action for health professionals. Chin Med J (Engl). 2020;133:1552–60.
10. Pawankar R, Wang JY, Wang IJ, et al. Asia Pacific Association of Allergy Asthma and Clinical Immunology White Paper 2020 on climate change, air pollution, and biodiversity in Asia-Pacific and impact on allergic diseases. Asia Pac Allergy 2020;10:e11.
11. Lu C, Liu Z, Yang W, et al. Early life exposure to outdoor air pollution and indoor environmental factors on the development of childhood allergy from early symptoms to diseases. Environ Res 2023;216(Pt 2):114538.
12. Fan HC, Chen CM, Tsai JD, et al. Association between Exposure to Particulate Matter Air Pollution during Early Childhood and Risk of Attention-Deficit/Hyperactivity Disorder in Taiwan. Int J Environ Res Public Health 2022;19:16138.

13. Mansouri A, Wei W, Alessandrini, et al. Impact of Climate Change on Indoor Air Quality: A Review. Int J Environ Res Public Health 2022;19(23):15616.
14. Brennan T. Indoor Environmental Quality and Climate Change. The Indoor Environments Division Office of Radiation and Indoor Air, U.S. Environmental Protection Agency; Available at: https://www.epa.gov/sites/default/files/2014-08/documents/climate_change_brennan.pdf. Accessed June 8, 2023.
15. Vardoulakis, S., Heaviside, C., (eds), 2012. Health Effects of Climate Change in the UK 2012; Current evidence, recommendations and research gaps. ISBN 978-0-85951-723-2. Health ProtectionAgency.Available at: https://assets.publishing.service.gov.uk/government/uploads/system/uploads/attachment_data/file/371103/Health_Effects_of_Climate_Change_in_the_UK_2012_V13_with_cover_accessible.pdf. Accessed June 8, 2023.
16. WHO. Air quality guidelines for Europe. 2nd edition. World Health Organization, Copenhagen WHO Regional Publications; 2000. European Series; 91. Air quality guidelines for Europe, 2nd edition (who.int).
17. D'Amato G, Liccardi G, D'Amato M, et al. Outdoor air pollution, climatic changes and allergic bronchial asthma. Eur Respir J 2002;20:763–76.
18. Solberg S, Hov Ø, Søvde A, et al. European surface ozone in the extreme summer 2003. J Geophys Res 2008;113:D07307.
19. Adetona O, Simpson CD, Li Z, et al. Hydroxylated polycyclic aromatic hydrocarbons as biomarkers of exposure to wood smoke in wildland frefghters. J Expo Sci Environ Epidemiol 2017;27:78–83.
20. Orecchio S, Amorello D, Barreca S, et al. Speciation of vanadium in urban, industrial, volcanic soils by a modifed Tessier method. Environmental Science: Process Impacts 2016;18:323–9.
21. O'Connor J, Mickan B, Siddique KH, et al. Physical, chemical, microbial contaminants in food waste management for soil application: a review. Environmental Pollution 2022;300:118860.
22. Zhong L, Su FC, Batterman S. Volatile organic compounds (VOCs) in conventional and high performance school buildings in the US. Int J Environ Res Public Health 2017b;14:100.
23. Vasile V, Petran H, Dima A, et al. Indoor air quality–a key element of the energy performance of the buildings. Energy Proc 2016;96:277–84.
24. Davidson CI, Phalen RF, Solomon PA. Airborne particulate matter, human health: a review. Aerosol Science. Technology 2005;39:737–49.
25. Teiri H, Hajizadeh Y, Azhdarpoor A. A review of different phytoremediation methods, critical factors for purification of common indoor air pollutants: an approach with sensitive analysis. Air Quality, Atmosphere & Health 2022;15:373–91.
26. Maisey SJ, Saunders SM, West N, et al. An extended baseline examination of indoor VOCs in a city of low ambient pollution: Perth, Western Australia. Atmos Environ 2013;81:546–53.
27. Trostl J, Herrmann E, Frege C, et al. Contribution of new particle formation to the total aerosol concentration at the high-altitude site Jungfraujoch (3580 m asl, Switzerland). J Geophys Res Atmos 2016;121:11–692.
28. Gonzalez-Martin J, Kraakman NJR, Perez C, et al. A state–of–the-art review on indoor air pollution, strategies for indoor air pollution control. Chemosphere 2021;262:128–376.
29. Yang L, Li C, Tang X. The Impact of PM2.5 on the Host Defense of Respiratory System. Front Cell Dev Biol 2020;8:91.
30. WHO Handbook on indoor Radon: a Public health perspective. Geneva: World Health Organization; 2009.

31. AGIR. Radon and Public Health. Report of the Advisory Group on Ionising radiation (HPARCE-11); 2009.
32. Mudarri D, Fisk WJ. Public health and economic impact of dampness and mold. Indoor Air 2007;17:226–35.
33. Gutarowska B, Piotrowska M. Methods of mycological analysis in buildings. Build Environ 2007;42:1843–50.
34. Trout D, Bernstein J, Martinez K, et al. Bioaerosol lung damage in a worker with repeated exposure to fungi in a water-damaged building. Environ Health Perspect 2001;109(6):641–4.
35. Gomes ML, Morais A, Cavaleiro Rufo J. The association between fungi exposure and hypersensitivity pneumonitis: a systematic review. Porto Biomed J 2021;6(1): e117.
36. Cheng KJ, Zhou ML, Liu YC, et al. Allergic fungal rhinosinusitis accompanied by allergic bronchopulmonary aspergillosis: A case report and literature review. World J Clin Cases 2019;7(22):3821–31.
37. Kennedy R, Smith M. Effects of aeroallergens on human health under climate change. In: Vardoulakis S, Heaviside C, editors. Health Effects of Climate Change in the UK. UK: Health Protection Agency; 2012. p. 83–91.
38. Katelaris CH, Beggs PJ. Climate change: allergens and allergic diseases. Intern Med J 2018;48:129–34.
39. D'Amato G, Annesi-Maesano I, Cecchi L, et al. Latest news on relationship between thunderstorms and respiratory allergy, severe asthma, and deaths for asthma. Allergy 2019;74:9–11.
40. Ferreira A, Barros N. COVID-19 and Lockdown: The Potential Impact of Residential Indoor Air Quality on the Health of Teleworkers. Int J Environ Res Public Health 2022;19:6079.
41. Gupta S, Rouse BT, Sarangi PP. Did Climate Change Influence the Emergence, Transmission, and Expression of the COVID-19 Pandemic? Front Med 2021;8: 769208.
42. Kitzberger T, Brown PM, Heyerdahl EK, et al. Contingent Pacific–Atlantic Ocean influence on multicentury wildfire synchrony over western North America. Proc Natl Acad Sci USA 2007;104(2):543–8.
43. U.S. EPA. An Office Building Occupant's Guide to Indoor Air Quality. Available at: http://www.epa.gov/iaq/pubs/occupgd.html. Accessed June 8, 2023.
44. U.S. Environmental Protection Agency. 1987. The total exposure assessment methodology (TEAM) study: Summary and analysis. EPA/600/6-87/002a. Washington, DC.
45. CDC. Healthy Housing Reference Manual. Chapter 5: Indoor Air Pollutants and Toxic Materials. Available at: http://www.cdc.gov/nceh/publications/books/housing/cha05.html. Accessed June 8, 2023.
46. American Society of Heating, Refrigerating and Air-Conditioning Engineers (ASHRAE) ASHRAE Standard 62.1. Ventilation for Acceptable Indoor Air Quality. 2010. Atlanta, GA.
47. A 2021 Guide to the Indoor Air Quality Standards that Matter. Available at: https://i-qlair.com/2021-guide-indoor-air-quality-standards. Accessed June 8, 2023.
48. Fuller GW, Tremper AH, Baker TD, et al. Contribution of wood burning to PM10 in London. Atmos Environ 2014;87:87–94.
49. Fuller S, Bulkeley H. Changing countries, changing climates: achieving thermal comfort through adaptation in everyday activities. Area 2013;45:63–9.

50. Vardoulakis S, Dimitroulopoulou C, Thornes J, et al. Impact of climate change on the domestic indoor environment and associated health risks in the UK. Environ Int 2015;85:299–313.
51. Beizaee A, Lomas KJ, Firth SK. National survey of summertime temperatures and overheating risk in English homes. Build Environ 2013;65:1–17.
52. Firth, S.K., Wright, A.J. Investigating the thermal characteristics of English dwellings: Summer temperatures. Air Conditioning and the Low Carbon Cooling Challenge. Network for Comfort and Energy Use in Buildings (NCEUB), 2008.Windsor, UK.
53. Chen J, Brager GS, Augenbroe G, et al. Impact of outdoor air quality on the natural ventilation usage of commercial buildings in the US. Appl Energy 2019;235: 673–84.
54. Wei S, Jones R, De Wilde P. Driving factors for occupant-controlled space heating in residential buildings. Energy and Buildings 2013;70:36–44.
55. Fauquert JL, Alba-Linero C, Gherasim A, et al. Organ-specific allergen challenges in airway allergy: Current utilities and future directions. Allergy 2023; 78(7):1794–809.
56. Colas C, Brosa M, Anton E, et al. Estimate of the total costs of allergic rhinitis in specialized care based on real-world data: the FERIN Study. Allergy 2017;72: 959–66.
57. Belhassen M, Demoly P, Bloch-Morot E, et al. Costs of perennial allergic rhinitis and allergic asthma increase with severity and poor disease control. Allergy 2017;72:948–58.
58. Bousquet J, Khaltaev N, Cruz AA, et al. Allergic rhinitis and its impact on asthma (ARIA) 2008 update (in collaboration with the World Health Organization, GA(2) LEN and AllerGen). Allergy 2008;63(Suppl 86):8–160.
59. Eguiluz-Gracia I, Mathioudakis AG, Bartel S, et al. The need for clean air: The way air pollution and climate change affect allergic rhinitis and asthma. Allergy 2020; 75:2170–84.
60. Hackett TL, Singhera GK, Shaheen F, et al. Intrinsic phenotypic differences of asthmatic epithelium and its inflammatory responses to respiratory syncytial virus and air pollution. Am J Respir Cell Mol Biol 2011;45:1090–100.
61. Brunekreef B, Von Mutius E, Wong G, et al. Exposure to cats and dogs, and symptoms of asthma, rhinoconjunctivitis, and eczema. Epidemiology 2012;23: 742–50.
62. Luczynska CM, Li Y, Chapman MD, et al. Airborne concentrations and particle size distribution of allergen derived from domestic cats (Felis domesticus). Measurements using cascade impactor, liquid impinger, and a two-site monoclonal antibody assay for Fel d 1. Am Rev Respir Dis 1990;141:361–7, 24.
63. Custovic A, Simpson A, Pahdi H, et al. Distribution, aerodynamic characteristics, and removal of the major cat allergen Fel d 1 in British homes. Thorax 1998; 53:33–8.
64. Ruggieri S, Drago G, Longo V, et al. Sensitization to dust mite defines different phenotypes of asthma: a multicenter study. Pediatr Allergy Immunol 2017;28: 675–82.
65. Ziello C, Sparks TH, Estrella N, et al. Changes to airborne pollen counts across Europe. PLoS One 2012;7:e34076.
66. Cakmak S, Dales RE, Coates F. Does air pollution increase the effect of aeroallergens on hospitalization for asthma. J Allergy Clin Immunol 2012;129:228–31.
67. Guilbert A, Cox B, Bruffaerts N, et al. Relationships between aeroallergen levels and hospital admissions for asthma in the Brussels-Capital Region: a daily time series analysis. Environ Health 2018;17:018–0378.

68. William J, Fisk BCS, Chan WR. Association of residential energy efficiency retrofits with indoor environmental quality, comfort, and health: A review of empirical data. Build Environ 2020;180:107067.

69. Gens A, Hurley JF, Tuomisto JT, et al. Health impacts due to personal exposure to fine particles caused by insulation of residential buildings in Europe. Atmos Environ 2014;84:213–21.

70. Gherasim A, de Blay F. Does Air Filtration Work for Cat Allergen Exposure? Curr Allergy Asthma Rep 2020;20:18.

71. Gherasim A, Jacob A, Schoettel F, et al. Efficacy of air cleaners in asthmatics allergic to cat in ALYATEC® environmental exposure chamber. Clin Exp Allergy 2020;50:160–9.

72. Singer BC, Chan WR, Kim YS, et al. Indoor air quality in California homes with code-required mechanical ventilation. Indoor Air 2020;30:885–99.

73. Balvers J, Bogers R, Jongeneel R, et al. Mechanical ventilation in recently built Dutch homes: technical shortcomings, possibilities for improvement, perceived indoor environment and health effects. Agricultural Science Review 2012; 55:4–14.

74. Laverge J, Janssens A. Carbon Dioxide Concentrations and Humidity Levels Measured in Belgian Standard and Low Energy Dwellings with Common Ventilation Strategies. Int J Vent 2015;14:165–80.

75. Cortez-Lugo M, Moreno-Macias H, Holguin-Molina, et al. Relationship between indoor, outdoor, and personal fine particle concentrations for individuals with COPD and predictors of indoor-outdoor ratio in Mexicocity. J Expo Sci Environ Epidemiol 2008;18:109–15.

76. Cortez-Lugo M, Ramirez-Aguilar M, Perez-Padilla R, et al. Effect of Personal Exposure to PM2.5 on Respiratory Health in a Mexican Panel of Patients with COPD. Int. J. Environ. Res. Public Health. 2015;12:10635–47.

77. Cleary E, Asher M, Olawoyin R, et al. Assessment of indoor air quality exposures and impacts on respiratory outcomes in River Rouge and Dearborn, Michigan. Chemosphere 2017;187:320–9.

78. Delfino RJ, Staimer N, Gillen D, et al. Personal and ambient air pollution is associated with increased exhaled nitric oxide in children with asthma. Environ Health Perspect 2006;114:1736–43.

79. Fang L, Norris C, Johnson K, et al. Toxic volatile organic compounds in 20 homes in Shanghai: Concentrations, inhalation health risks, and the impacts of household air cleaning. Build Environ 2019;157:309–18.

80. Jansen KL, Larson TV, Koenig JQ, et al. Associations between health effects and particulate matter and black carbon in subjects with respiratory disease. Environ Health Perspect 2005;113:1741–6.

81. Kearney J, Wallace L, MacNeil M, et al. Residential indoor and outdoor ultrafine particles in Windsor, Ontario. Atmos Environ 2011;45:7583–93.

82. Rojas-Bracho L, Suh H, Koutrakis P. Relationships among personal, indoor, and outdoor fine and coarse particle concentrations for individuals with COPD. J Expo Anal Environ Epidemiol 2000;10:294–306.

83. Soppa VJ, Schins RP, Henning F, et al. Respiratory Effects of Fine and Ultrafine Particles from Indoor Sources—A Randomized Sham-Controlled Exposure Study of Healthy Volunteers. Int. J. Environ. Res. Public Health. 2014;11:6871–89.

84. Trenga CA, Sullivan JH, Schildcrout, et al. Effect of particulate air, pollution on lung function in adult and paediatric subjects in a Seattle panel study. Chest 2006;129:1614–22.

85. Vardoulakis S, Giagloglou E, Steinle S, et al. Indoor Exposure to Selected Air Pollutants in the Home Environment: A Systematic Review. Int. J. Environ. Res. Public Health 2020;17:8972.
86. Weichenthal S, Dufresne A, Infanate-Rivard C. Indoor nitrogen dioxide and VOC exposures: Summary of evidence for an association with childhood asthma and a case for the inclusion of indoor ultrafine particle measures in future studies. Indoor Built Environ 2008;16:387–99.
87. Xia X, Qiu H, Kwok T, et al. Time course of blood oxygen saturation responding to short-term fine particulate matter among elderly healthy subjects and patients with chronic obstructive pulmonary disease. Sci Total Environ 2020;723:138022.
88. Bernstein JA, Bobbitt RC, Levin L, et al. Health effects of ultraviolet irradiation in asthmatic children's homes. J Asthma 2006;43(4):255–62.
89. Han KT, Ruan LW. Effects of indoor plants on air quality: a systematic review. Environ Sci Pollut Res 2020;27:16019–51.
90. Cruz MD, Tomasi G, Müller R, et al. Removal of volatile gasoline compounds by indoor potted plants studied by pixel-based fingerprinting analysis. Chemosphere 2019;221:226–34.
91. Kubesch NJ, Therming Jorgensen J, Hoffmann B, et al. Effects of leisure-time and transport-related physical activities on the risk of incident and recurrent myocardial infarction and interaction with traffic-related air Pollution: a Cohort Study. J Am Heart Assoc 2018;7–15.
92. Erbas B, Jazayeri M, Lambert KA, et al. Outdoor pollen is a trigger of child and adolescent asthma emergency department presentations: A systematic review and meta-analysis. Allergy 2018;73:1632–41.
93. Bousquet J, Caimmi DP, Bedbrook A, et al. Pilot study of mobile phone technology in allergic rhinitis in European countries: the MASK-rhinitis study. Allergy 2017;72:857–65, 178.
94. European Union's (EU) 2050 Climate strategies and target: Low carbon Economy. Available at: https://ec.europa.eu/clima/policies/strategies/2050_en. Accessed July 1, 2018.
95. Giorgi F, Meleux F. Modelling the regional effects of climate change on air quality. C. R. Geosci. 2007;339:721–33.
96. Cao Y, Yue X, Liao H, et al. Ensemble projection of global isoprene emissions by the end of 21st century using CMIP6 models. Atmos Environ 2021;267:118766.
97. Jutel M, Mosnaim GS, Bernstein JA, et al. The One Health approach for allergic diseases and asthma. Allergy 2023;78(7):1777–93.
98. Costello A, Abbas M, Allen A, et al. Managing the health effects of climate change: Lancet and University College London Institute for Global Health Commission. Lancet 2009;373:1693–733.

Climate Change and Food Allergy

Ashley Sang Eun Lee, MD[a,b,*], Nicole Ramsey, MD, PhD[a,b]

KEYWORDS

- Climate change • Global warming • Greenhouse gases • Food allergy
- Oral allergy syndrome • Eosinophilic esophagitis

KEY POINTS

- The role of climate change and consequent influences of air pollution on food allergy remains less explored compared with impacts on allergic rhinitis and asthma.
- In this review, we discuss the epithelial barrier hypothesis as a proposed mechanism of food allergy development that may be relevant in this context.
- We discuss existing studies that provide insight into the intricate relationship between food allergy and climate-related environmental factors.

INTRODUCTION

Food allergy affects 8% of children and 10% of adults in the United States, with its prevalence increasing in the United States and other parts of the world, including Africa and Asia, especially in urban areas.[1–3] The relationship between climate change and food allergy remains less explored in comparison to other allergic disorders such as rhinitis and asthma.[4] However, the increased prevalence of food allergy In the setting of industrialization suggests that environmental exposures including temperature changes and increased air pollutants such as particulate matter (PM), carbon dioxide (CO_2), and ozone (O_3) may be contributory.[5] In this review, we discuss the epithelial barrier hypothesis as a proposed mechanism of the increased development of food allergy in the setting of climate change, as well as the effect of anthropogenic emissions on pollination patterns, thereby affecting pollen food allergy syndrome (PFAS), peanut (the most common food allergen), and non-immunoglobulin E- mediated food allergic conditions such as eosinophilic esophagitis (EoE).

[a] Division of Allergy and Immunology, Icahn School of Medicine at Mount Sinai, 1425 Madison Avenue, New York 10029, USA; [b] Department of Pediatrics, Jaffe Food Allergy Institute, 10540 Avenue K, Brooklyn, NY 11236-3018, USA
* Corresponding author. 1425 Madison Ave, 11th floor, New York, NY 10029.
E-mail address: ashleysangeun.lee@mssm.edu

Immunol Allergy Clin N Am 44 (2024) 75–83
https://doi.org/10.1016/j.iac.2023.07.003
0889-8561/24/© 2023 Elsevier Inc. All rights reserved.
immunology.theclinics.com

THE EPITHELIAL BARRIER HYPOTHESIS, IMMUNOGLOBULIN E SENSITIZATION, AND FOOD ALLERGY HISTORY

The epithelial barrier hypothesis (**Fig. 1**) has been proposed to account for the association between industrialization and the increased prevalence of allergic diseases, including food allergy.[5] Based on the epithelial barrier hypothesis, exposure to environmental toxins disrupts the integrity of the epithelial barrier in various organs, including the skin, gut, and airway.[5] Disruption of the epithelial barrier not only allows for increased sensitization to environmental and food allergens but also introduces opportunistic pathogens and tissue inflammation.[6] Overlapping lines of research provide proof of concept that epithelial barrier disruption may be an underlying mechanism linking climate-related factors to food allergy trends. Mouse studies using mycotoxigenic fungi, an adjuvant thought to be increased in prevalence due to climate change, have demonstrated an association between epithelial barrier dysfunction and food allergy model severity.[6]

Fluctuations in global temperature and CO_2 levels have been proposed to influence the degree of mycotoxigenic fungi contamination of crops.[7] In a mouse model study, Drønen and colleagues showed that dietary mycotoxin deoxynivalenol (DON), a mycotoxigenic fungi found on grains including maize, barley, and wheat,[8] may act as an adjuvant in the development of peanut allergy.[9] Previous data from mouse models have shown that DON has adjuvant capacities of promoting food allergy by impairing mucosal integrity and function, which may lead to a leaky gut with increased uptake of allergens.[6,10] In addition, gut mucosal barriers can produce a subset of pro-Th2 (t helper 2) cytokines, such as interleukin (IL) 33 and thymic stromal lymphopoietin (TSLP) in response to external environmental toxins, a process that subsequently leads

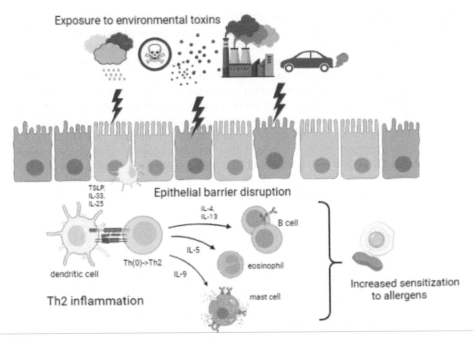

Fig. 1. Effect of environmental toxins and climate change on the epithelial barrier: environmental toxins including particular matter and CO_2 can damage the epithelial barrier, increasing the risk of sensitization to food allergens. (Created with BioRender.com.)

to the production of Th-2 cytokines by innate immune cells.[11] In the study published by Drønen and colleagues, mice exposed to DON and peanut had increased anaphylaxis scores, as measured by lower body temperature and increased presence of serum mast cell protease, compared with controls.[9] Mice exposed to DON, with or without coexposure to peanuts, also had early, short-term elevation of pro-Th2 inflammatory cytokines such as IL-33 and TSLP in the intestinal tissue, and the IL-33 receptor ST2 in the serum. Stimulated cells from these mice released additional inflammatory cytokines such as tumor necrosis factor-alpha, IL-6, and interferon-gamma. These results suggest DON induces an early-stage inflammation in the gut, which may predispose mice to increased uptake and sensitization to peanut allergens.[10,11]

Another mouse study by Seyed Toutounchi and colleagues, showed DON's role as an adjuvant that could prenatally predispose offspring to develop egg allergy.[12] Upon exposure to ovalbumin, mice born from mothers with a DON-contaminated diet had increased acute allergic skin response and elevated serum IgE, IgG1, and IgG2 to ovalbumin, compared with offspring born from mothers without a DON-contaminated diet. Furthermore, mice with egg allergy and prenatal DON exposure had a lower splenic T-regulatory cell population than those with egg allergy without prenatal DON exposure.[12]

While data from animal studies suggest environmental exposures can disrupt the epithelial barrier and thereby increase allergic sensitization to peanut or egg, there is a lack of consistent data in humans. For instance, a large Chinese cohort study of 2598 children showed that children aged 3 to 4 years who were exposed to outdoor pollution, particularly nitrogen dioxide (NO_2) had an increased prevalence of food allergy.[13] These findings highlight the role of airway epithelium in IgE-mediated food allergy, thereby supporting the epithelial barrier hypothesis.[13] Analysis of a separate cohort in the Netherlands (the Prevention and Incidence of Asthma and Mite Allergy cohort) showed that long-term exposure to PM2.5, soot, and NO_2 was associated with an increased risk of sensitization to food allergens by 4 years of age.[14] However, data from 4 European cohorts (part of the Mechanisms of the Development of Allergy consortium) consisting of 6163 children under the age of 16 years showed no clear association between air pollution (as measured by elevated PM2.5, PM10, and NO2 levels) and IgE-sensitization to food allergens.[15] Such variance in findings may be due to several factors including measurement approaches, geographic covariants, and exposure to pollutants with varying relative contributions. First, there are different techniques for measuring air pollution exposure with different sensitivities, including spot testing methods and machine learning methods. Some examples are open-path Fourier-transform infrared spectroscopy, which detects particles in the atmosphere, as well as quantum cascade laser open-path system, and tunable laser absorption spectroscope.[16] More recently, machine learning models have been used more frequently for air pollution detection; however, validation of data is needed for this method to ensure accuracy.[16] Second, air pollution can be measured via fixed environmental sensors or continuous mobile sensors.[17,18] Unlike fixed sensors that are deployed at specific monitoring sites, mobile sensors allow for the measurement of finer spatiotemporal resolution across various buildings, neighborhoods, and cities.[17,18] Third, temperature itself may be a contributing factor to the variability of air pollution levels. For instance, Jarvi and colleagues found that according to mobile laboratory and drone-measured levels of air pollutants including nitric oxide, O_3, and aerosol particles, thermal turbulence was associated with the formation of aerosol particle hotspots in winter, and that vertical decay was controlled mostly by the air temperature.[19] Finally, secondary pollutants may arise from additional sources of pollution and the effect of exposure to primary and secondary pollution sources with relative contribution may vary by geographic location. For example, emission regulations have led to an overall decrease in volatile organic compounds (VOCs), but other emission sources such as evaporative emission from volatile consumer products have led to an increase in intermediate VOCs, which also contributes to O_3 formation.[20] Wang and colleagues showed that independent of temperature changes, PM2.5 levels in the suburban district in Shanghai were higher than the urban level and that new particulate formation to cloud condensation nuclei (secondary pollutants) may be higher in urban areas compared with rural areas in China.[21]

THE EFFECT OF CLIMATE CHANGE ON IgE-MEDIATED FOOD ALLERGY: POLLEN FOOD ALLERGY SYNDROME

The epithelial barrier hypothesis may account for why some patients with environmental allergies develop PFAS, and how these patients may be at additional risk in the setting of climate change. Climate change (and increasing CO_2 levels) are projected to affect pollination patterns across the globe.[22]

Multiple food allergens including fruits, vegetables, legumes, and tree nuts are cross-reactive with pollen, thereby causing mild symptoms in patients with allergic rhinitis. These symptoms are consistent with PFAS, a type of IgE-mediated food allergy that affects 47% to 70% of individuals with allergic rhinitis.[23] PFAS results in mild oropharyngeal symptoms such as mouth and throat itching, about 5 to 15 minutes after ingestion of the culprit food. Symptoms are usually transient and resolve in 30 minutes,[24] but symptoms of PFAS may be worse at peak pollen seasons, and anaphylaxis can occur in up to 1.7% of patients.[23]

Birch pollen, a major culprit of spring allergies, is cross-reactive with multiple foods. Patients with birch (allergen Bet v1) sensitization may experience symptoms of PFAS after consuming food containing homologous proteins to Bet v1, including pitted fruits such as apricot, plum, cherry; vegetables such as carrot, celery, and parsley; legumes such as soy and peanut, and tree nuts such as almond and hazelnut.[23] The allergenic proteins in these foods are heat-labile and denatured by heating, cooking, and/or processing. Patients with ragweed allergy (allergen Amb a 1[25]), a major fall allergen, may experience PFAS symptoms after ingesting raw banana, melon, peach, and kiwi.[23]

On the basis of the existing data, it is expected that climate change may lead to an increase of pollination in various parts of the world,[22] thereby worsening symptoms for those with PFAS. Prior studies suggest pollen quantity and allergenicity are affected by changes in temperature and CO_2 levels.[22] For example, integrative modeling studies have shown that climate change resulting from anthropometric emissions may lead to fluctuations in birch pollination patterns in Central Europe.[22] It is also projected that birch allergy may become more common in areas of higher altitude, as birch trees may become more abundant in these areas.[22]

Wan and colleagues have shown that experimental warming significantly increases the pollen diameter and total production of Western ragweed (Ambrosia psilostachya).[26] In addition, environmental aeroallergen monitoring studies have noted atmospheric increases in ragweed pollen concentration in the twentieth century. For instance, a positive correlation between CO_2 levels and concentration of Amb a 1, a major ragweed allergen, has been noted in the past.[25] As CO_2 levels are expected to increase in the future, it is also expected that concentrations of Amb a 1 will increase even more.[25]

THE EFFECT OF CLIMATE CHANGE ON FOOD ALLERGEN: PEANUT

Peanut allergy is the most common type of food allergy in the United States, affecting about 2% of the population.[27] Classic IgE-mediated symptoms include hives/itching, oropharyngeal swelling, coughing, and/or vomiting within 30 minutes to 1 hour of exposure. Unfortunately, peanut allergy is rather persistent, with only 20% outgrowing their allergy in childhood.[28] In 2008, Beggs and Walczyk showed for the first time that increased temperature and CO_2 may impact allergenicity of the peanut plant (*Arachis hypogaea* L.).[29] Elevated CO_2 levels were associated with increased leaf photosynthesis, pollen viability, seed size, and shelling percentage, as well as decreased seed yield, seed set, and seed number per pod.[30,31] Increased temperature was associated with decreased flower production and number of pods per plant.[30,32] Changes in various characteristics of the peanut plant may imply fluctuations in the concentration of allergenic peanut proteins (Ara h1, 2, 3 which are different from Ara h8, a peanut allergen that is associated with PFAS), although data regarding this are scarce. More recently, however, Ziska and colleagues have shown that increased CO_2 levels are associated with an increase in Ara h1 (primary seed storage protein in peanuts, also a major allergen as mentioned above) levels.[32] Two types of peanut cultivars, Georgia Green (GA) and Virginia Jumbo (VA), were grown in 2 conditions, ambient and elevated CO_2 (ambient + 250 μmol mol^{-1} CO_2), for a 2 year period from 2012 to 2013. VA grown in hypercarbic conditions showed a consistently greater increase in above-ground biomass, seed yield, and Ara h1 levels in this 2 year period than VA grown in ambient conditions. GA grown in a hypercarbic environment had increased seed yield and above-ground biomass levels in 2013, and elevated Ara h1 levels in 2012, compared with GA grown in ambient conditions. Interestingly, the increase in Ara h1 levels in VA was negatively correlated with overall protein concentration.[32]

CLIMATE CHANGE AND THE ATOPIC MARCH

It is anticipated that climate change will lead to an increased incidence of atopic diseases.[4] The atopic march concept, which indicates those diagnosed with eczema are more likely to develop asthma, rhinitis, and/or food allergy later in life,[33] will also be a contributor to the increased incidence of allergic diseases in general. While an association between climate change and increased eczema and/or asthma incidence has been well established,[4] there are less data on food allergy. Interestingly, asthma is a risk factor for the development of food allergy, and food allergy is a risk factor for allergic asthma, especially if one is sensitized to a food allergen within the first few years of life.[34] The coexistence of both conditions increases the risk of food-related anaphylaxis and life-threatening asthma exacerbations.[34] For instance, a study of 88 children with cow's milk allergy showed that children with asthma had 10 times the number of severe reactions to accidental milk ingestion compared with milk-allergic children without asthma.[35]

THE EFFECT OF CLIMATE CHANGE ON NON-IgE-MEDIATED FOOD ALLERGIC CONDITION: EOSINOPHILIC ESOPHAGITIS

EoE is a non-IgE-mediated clinicopathologic disorder of the esophageal tract leading to esophageal dysfunction without appropriate treatment. A diagnosis of EoE requires clinical symptoms including abdominal pain, dysphagia, and failure to thrive (often seen in infants), as well as esophageal pathology consisting of at least 15 eosinophils per high-power field.[36] Studies suggest that there is an association between aeroallergen sensitization and EoE exacerbations.[37,38] For example, a large cross-sectional study of esophageal biopsies at the University of North Carolina hospitals showed that biopsies of patients who experienced exacerbation of EoE symptoms at peak pollen seasons were more severe than those who did not experience seasonal flares.[38] Esophageal rings, furrows, and strictures were seen more frequently in the tissues of patients with seasonal flares. Patients with seasonal flares also had worsening Endoscopic Reference Scores, evidenced by significant edema, furrows, and exudates compared with their pre-endoscopic findings.[38]

Onbasi and colleagues suggest that climate change and anthropogenic emissions may be associated with EoE.[37] This case-crossover study of EoE patients who presented to the emergency room in Utah showed that exposure to air pollution (as measured by PM2.5) increased the odds of food impaction by more than 5 fold.[37] A possible mechanism for this association is damage to the tight junction proteins of the esophageal epithelium, leading to increased exposure to reactive oxidative species induced by PM2.5.[39–41] As climate change and anthropomorphic emissions are expected to alter pollination patterns across the globe, the disease burden of EoE may increase in association.

In addition, Jensen and Dellon report an association between the risk of EoE diagnosis and climate zones.[42] Based on a national pathology database consisting of 14,381 EoE cases and 89,754 controls, patients living in cold climate zones had a 40% increased risk of being diagnosed with EoE compared with those living in warmer climate zones. The authors postulate that climate zones will affect local vegetation patterns and thereby aeroallergen exposure, which has been linked with EoE flares. A cross-sectional study using the same aforementioned database examined the relationship between EoE and seasonal patterns. Late spring and summer months were associated with higher odds of esophageal biopsies with 15 or greater eosinophils/HPF.[43] In addition, greater seasonal variation was seen in temperate and cooler climates, which may lead to more seasonality "peaks" than in dry or tropical climates.

CHALLENGES TO RESEARCH LINKING CLIMATE-RELATED FACTORS AND FOOD ALLERGY

Further long-term studies are needed to establish a clear relationship between climate change and food allergy trends over time. A barrier to understanding the described pattern is distinguishing allergen sensitization from clinical reactivity. For instance, although elevated levels in component or specific IgE levels may increase the rate of food sensitization in a population, this does not necessarily suggest clinical reactivity. The gold standard for a definitive diagnosis of food allergy requires a physician-supervised food challenge, which carries logistical and ethical challenges for prospective studies. In addition, pollination patterns vary across the world and are dependent on several factors, including deforestation, which will inevitably affect pollen counts. It is also worth noting that many population studies discussed in this review were derived from non-US cohorts, which implies the exposure profile of these patients may not be applicable to those in the United States.

SUMMARY

Following the industrialization era, there has been a drastic increase in the prevalence of food allergy throughout the world. Prior research suggests that the detrimental sequelae of industrialization, including anthropogenic emissions and climate change, are contributory to the increase in the prevalence of food allergy. The mechanism by which this association occurs may in part be explained by the epithelial barrier hypothesis—various environmental exposures such as mycotoxigenic fungi, PM, and CO_2, compromising the integrity of the epithelial barrier in the skin, airway, and gut, leading to increased sensitization and inflammation that may increase an individual's risk of developing food allergy. Climate change is also projected to increase pollination patterns in various parts of the world, with existing studies suggestive of impending increases of birch (spring allergen) and ragweed (fall) allergens, which may increase the incidence of PFAS and potentially worsen symptom severity for those already affected by PFAS. Similarly, those with EoE may have increased EoE exacerbations as pollen counts increase. The incidence of peanut allergy and/or sensitization may increase with air pollution, as Ara h1 levels are expected to increase with atmospheric CO_2 levels. Overall, we anticipate that climate change and air pollutants will increase the incidence of food allergic disorders and carry significant consequences including compromised quality of life of those affected by these disorders, as well as increased health care utilization. Additional mechanistic and longitudinal studies are needed to better understand the complex dynamic relationships between climate change and food allergy.

CLINICS CARE POINTS

- Environmental exposures such as mycotoxigenic fungi and anthropogenic emissions may disrupt the epithelial barrier, increasing the risk of food allergen sensitization.
- Pollination patterns are expected to affect various food allergy disorders, including PFAS, peanut allergy, and EoE.
- There is a need for additional long-term studies to further characterize the association between climate change and food allergy.

DISCLOSURE

The authors have nothing to disclose.

REFERENCES

1. Warren CM, Jiang J, Gupta RS. Epidemiology and Burden of Food Allergy. Curr Allergyasthma Rep 2020;20(2):6.
2. Peters RL, Krawiec M, Koplin JJ, et al. Update on food allergy. In: Ebisawa M, editor. Pediatr Allergy Immunol 2021;32(4):647–57.
3. Gupta RS, Warren CM, Smith BM, et al. Prevalence and Severity of Food Allergies Among US Adults. JAMA Netw Open 2019;2(1):e185630.
4. Celebi Sozener Z, Ozdel Ozturk B, Cerci P, et al. Epithelial barrier hypothesis: Effect of the external exposome on the microbiome and epithelial barriers in allergic disease. Allergy 2022;77(5):1418–49.
5. Akdis CA. Does the epithelial barrier hypothesis explain the increase in allergy, autoimmunity and other chronic conditions? Nat Rev Immunol 2021;21(11): 739–51.
6. Akdis CA. The epithelial barrier hypothesis proposes a comprehensive understanding of the origins of allergic and other chronic noncommunicable diseases. J Allergy Clin Immunol 2022;149(1):41–4.
7. Van der Fels-Klerx HJ, van Asselt ED, Madsen MS, et al. Impact of climate change effects on contamination of cereal grains with deoxynivalenol. PLoS ONE 2013;8(9):e73602.
8. Sumarah MW. The Deoxynivalenol Challenge. J Agric Food Chem 2022;70(31): 9619–24.
9. Drønen EK, Namork E, Dirven H, et al. Suspected gut barrier disruptors and development of food allergy: Adjuvant effects and early immune responses. Front Allergy 2022;3:1029125.

10. Smith PK, Masilamani M, Li XM, et al. The false alarm hypothesis: Food allergy is associated with high dietary advanced glycation end-products and proglycating dietary sugars that mimic alarmins. J Allergy Clin Immunol 2017;139(2):429–37.

11. Ramsey N, Berin MC. Pathogenesis of IgE-mediated food allergy and implications for future immunotherapeutics. Pediatr Allergy Immunol 2021;32(7): 1416–25.

12. Seyed Toutounchi N, Braber S, van't Land B, et al. Exposure to Deoxynivalenol During Pregnancy and Lactation Enhances Food Allergy and Reduces Vaccine Responsiveness in the Offspring in a Mouse Model. Front Immunol 2021;12: 797152.

13. Zhang X, Lu C, Li Y, et al. Early-life exposure to air pollution associated with food allergy in children: Implications for 'one allergy' concept. Environ Res 2023;216: 114713.

14. Brauer M, Hoek G, Smit HA, et al. Air pollution and development of asthma, allergy and infections in a birth cohort. Eur Respir J 2007;29(5):879–88.

15. Peters RL, Mavoa S, Koplin JJ. An Overview of Environmental Risk Factors for Food Allergy. Int J Environ Res Public Health 2022;19(2):722.

16. Mukundan A, Huang C-C, Men T-C, et al. Air Pollution Detection Using a Novel Snap-Shot Hyperspectral Imaging Technique. Sensors 2022;22(16):6231.

17. Singla S, Bansal D, Misra A, et al. Towards an integrated framework for air quality monitoring and exposure estimation-a review. Environ Monit Assess 2018; 190(9):562.

18. Shakhov V, Materukhin A, Sokolova O, et al. Optimizing Urban Air Pollution Detection Systems. Sensors 2022;22(13):4767.

19. Järvi L, Kurppa M, Kuuluvainen H, et al. Determinants of spatial variability of air pollutant concentrations in a street canyon network measured using a mobile laboratory and a drone. Sci Total Environ 2023;856(Pt 1):158974.

20. Drozd GT, Weber RJ, Goldstein AH. Highly Resolved Composition during Diesel Evaporation with Modeled Ozone and Secondary Aerosol Formation: Insights into Pollutant Formation from Evaporative Intermediate Volatility Organic Compound Sources. Environ Sci Technol 2021;55(9):5742–51.

21. Wang J, Zhao B, Wang S, et al. Particulate matter pollution over China and the effects of control policies. Sci Total Environ 2017;584-585:426–47.

22. Rojo J, Oteros J, Picornell A, et al. Effects of future climate change on birch abundance and their pollen load. Glob Change Biol 2021;27(22):5934–49.

23. Skypala IJ. Can patients with oral allergy syndrome be at risk of anaphylaxis? Curr Opin Allergy Clin Immunol 2020;20(5):459–64.

24. Carlson G, Coop C. Pollen food allergy syndrome (PFAS): A review of current available literature. Ann Allergy Asthma Immunol 2019;123(4):359–65.

25. Singer BD, Ziska LH, Frenz DA, et al. Research note: Increasing Amb a 1 content in common ragweed (Ambrosia artemisiifolia) pollen as a function of rising atmospheric CO2 concentration. Funct Plant Biol 2005;32(7):667.

26. Wan S, Yuan T, Bowdish S, et al. Response of an allergenic species, Ambrosia psilostachya (Asteraceae), to experimental warming and clipping: implications for public health. Am J Bot 2002;89(11):1843–6.

27. Thomas NM. Racial and Ethnic Data Reported for Peanut Allergy Epidemiology Do Little to Advance Its Cause, Treatment, or Prevention. Front Public Health 2021;9:685240.

28. Fleischer DM, Conover-Walker MK, Matsui EC, et al. The natural history of tree nut allergy. J Allergy Clin Immunol 2005;116(5):1087–93.

29. Beggs PJ, Walczyk NE. Impacts of climate change on plant food allergens: a previously unrecognized threat to human health. Air Qual Atmosphere Health 2008; 1(2):119–23.
30. Vu JCV. Acclimation of peanut (Arachis hypogaea L.) leaf photosynthesis to elevated growth CO2 and temperature. Environ Exp Bot 2005;53(1):85–95.
31. Vara Prasad PV, Craufurd PQ, Summerfield RJ, et al. Effects of short episodes of heat stress on flower production and fruit-set of groundnut (Arachis hypogaea L.). J Exp Bot 2000;51(345):777–84.
32. Ziska LH, Yang J, Tomecek MB, Beggs PJ. Cultivar-specific changes in peanut yield, biomass, and allergenicity in response to elevated atmospheric carbon dioxide concentration. Crop Science 2016;56(5):2766–74.
33. Luschkova D, Zeiser K, Ludwig A, et al. Atopic eczema is an environmentaldisease. Allergol Select 2021;5:244–50.
34. di Palmo E, Gallucci M, Cipriani F, et al. Asthma and Food Allergy: Which Risks? Medicina 2019;55(9):509.
35. Boyano-Martínez T, García-Ara C, Pedrosa M, et al. Accidental allergic reactions in children allergic to cow's milk proteins. J Allergy Clin Immunol 2009;123(4): 883–8.
36. Gonsalves NP, Aceves SS. Diagnosis and treatment of eosinophilic esophagitis. J Allergy Clin Immunol 2020;145(1):1–7.
37. Onbasi K, Sin AZ, Doganavsargil B, et al. Eosinophil infiltration of the oesophageal mucosa in patients with pollen allergy during the season. Clin Htmlent Glyphamp Asciiamp Exp Allergy 2005;35(11):1423–31.
38. Cianferoni A, Jensen E, Davis CM. The Role of the Environment in Eosinophilic Esophagitis. J Allergy Clin Immunol Pract 2021;9(9):3268–74.
39. May Maestas M, Perry KD, Smith K, et al. Food impactions in Eosinophilic esophagitis and acute exposures to fine particulate pollution. Allergy 2019;74(12): 2529–30.
40. Celebi Sözener Z, Cevhertas L, Nadeau K, et al. Environmental factors in epithelial barrier dysfunction. J Allergy Clin Immunol 2020;145(6):1517–28.
41. Piao MJ, Ahn MJ, Kang KA, et al. Particulate matter 2.5 damages skin cells by inducing oxidative stress, subcellular organelle dysfunction, and apoptosis. Arch Toxicol 2018;92:2077–91.
42. Jensen ET, Dellon ES. Environmental factors and eosinophilic esophagitis. J Allergy Clin Immunol 2018;142(1):32–40.
43. Jensen ET, Shah ND, Hoffman K, et al. Seasonal variation in detection of oesophageal eosinophilia and eosinophilic oesophagitis. Aliment Pharmacol Ther 2015;42(4):461–9.

Impact of Climate Change on Dietary Nutritional Quality and Implications for Asthma and Allergy

Kecia N. Carroll, MD, MPH

KEYWORDS

- Asthma • Allergic disorders • Climate change • Prenatal • Nutrition
- Long-chain polyunsaturated fatty acids • Antioxidants • Children

KEY POINTS

- Asthma and allergic disorders are common in childhood with environmental determinants of disease that include prenatal nutritional exposures such as long-chain polyunsaturated fatty acids (LC-PUFA) and antioxidants.
- Global climate change is implicated in asthma and allergic disorders and effects on aquatic and agricultural ecosystems may influence the availability and quality of LC-PUFAs and dietary antioxidants, respectively.
- In efforts to prevent or lessen the severity of asthma and allergic conditions, it is important to better understand the multiple mechanisms through which climate change may influence respiratory health, including impact on diverse ecosystems and associated food supply.

INTRODUCTION

Asthma and allergic disorders are common conditions in childhood[1-4] and are associated with significant clinical and psychosocial morbidity and consequent substantial health care utilization and costs.[5-8] Asthma and related allergic disorders are complex diseases with multiple genetic and environmental contributors.[9-14] The effects of global climate change are increasingly documented in relation to the expression of asthma and allergic conditions.[4,14-18] Although the impact of climate change on asthma and atopic conditions may be mediated through consequent alterations in a host of prenatal and postnatal ambient environmental triggers and allergens, climate change also influences the structure and composition of ecologic systems that may

Division of General Pediatrics, Departments of Pediatrics and Environmental Medicine & Public Health, Icahn School of Medicine at Mount Sinai, One Gustave L. Levy Place, Box 1198, New York, NY 10029, USA
E-mail address: Kecia.carroll@mssm.edu

Immunol Allergy Clin N Am 44 (2024) 85–96
https://doi.org/10.1016/j.iac.2023.09.002
0889-8561/24/© 2023 Elsevier Inc. All rights reserved.

have downstream impacts on the quality and availability of certain nutritional exposures.[15,19-21] Prenatal and early-life nutritional exposures have the potential to influence asthma and atopic disease development through effects on the developing immune system.[10,22-24] Climate effects such as increased ambient and ocean temperatures, increased carbon dioxide levels, and increased ocean acidification may adversely affect polyunsaturated fatty acid (PUFA)[19,21] and dietary antioxidant[25,26] availability which are two of the most extensively studied groups of micronutrients in relation to wheeze, asthma, and related allergic outcomes.[11,27-37] For example, omega-3 (n-3) and omega-6 (n-6) PUFAs are involved in the synthesis of proinflammatory and less inflammatory mediators, respectively, thus factors that influence prenatal intake of these nutritional exposures have the potential to influence the development of conditions such as asthma and allergic disorders.[19,38-40] Oxidative stress (OS) resulting from an imbalance between reactive oxygen species (ROS) and antioxidant defenses, is increasingly thought to play a central role in lung pathogenesis and asthma development.[41,42] This overview summarizes the role of these micronutrients in respiratory and related allergic disorders and briefly discusses how climate change can impact dietary quality specific to these factors.

Asthma Epidemiology: Role of Prenatal Nutritional Factors

Asthma is an inflammatory disease of the airways with genetic and environmental contributions[9,10] that is characterized by airway hyperresponsiveness, inflammation, and obstruction that is reversible, at least in part.[2] An estimated 6 million children in the United States are affected by asthma and there is substantial burden globally.[2,3] In addition, there are differences in asthma incidence and severity by sociodemographic exposures such as race/ethnicity and economic status with children from non-Hispanic black, specific Hispanic ethnicities, and lower-income backgrounds disproportionately affected.[43,44] Prenatal and early-life nutritional exposures have been linked with asthma and allergy-related conditions in childhood as well as changes in the developing immune system that highlight potential underlying pathophysiology including immune function alterations in cord blood associated with maternal prenatal n-3 PUFA supplementation.[24,45-48]

Long-Chain Polyunsaturated Fatty Acids

PUFAs are bioactive compounds that are involved in several biologic processes.[49,50] The n-3 and n-6 PUFA series have 18 or more carbon atoms and one classification is based on the number of carbon atoms, number of double bonds, and the location of the first double bond counting from the omega end of the compound.[49,50] PUFAs in the n-3 PUFA series from marine sources are primarily eicosapentaenoic acid (EPA) and docosahexaenoic acid (DHA) while plant-based oils, seeds, and nuts are sources of alpha-linolenic acid (ALA). PUFAs in the n-6 series are consumed primarily from plant-based oils and seeds, linoleic acid (LA), in addition to red meats, arachidonic acid (AA), or marine-based sources, docosapentaenoic acid. PUFAs are incorporated into cell membrane phospholipids and are involved in the synthesis of inflammatory mediators including prostaglandins, leukotrienes, and thromboxanes.[39,50]

Omega-3 and n-6 PUFAs have potentially opposing biologic activity as regards to inflammation.[24] AA, an n-6 PUFA derived from LA, is typically the most abundant LC-PUFA in cell membranes and when released from cells serves as substrate for bioactive lipid mediators including prostaglandins and thromboxanes or leukotrienes generated from cyclooxygenase or lipoxygenase pathways, respectively.[24] Although prostaglandin E_2 has anti-inflammatory activities, it also promotes allergic inflammation including IgE production. In addition, AA derivative PGD_2 and leukotriene B_4 are involved in the production of Th2-type and pro-inflammatory cytokines from immune cells.[39,51–54] N3 LC-PUFAs have opposing functions as they may replace AA in cell membranes with resultant decrease in n-6 LC-PUFA activity. This is particularly relevant as prostaglandins and thromboxanes produced from the EPA are associated with less inflammatory profiles than AA[24,39,40,55–57] and EPA and DHA are also converted to resolvins which play a role in the resolution of inflammation. Omega-3 and n-6 PUFA dietary intakes may influence cell membrane composition and furthermore n-3 and n-6 PUFAs compete for the same enzymes (eg, elongase and desaturase) in biological processes that involve conversion of ALA and LA to downstream n-3 and n-6 long-chain (LC) PUFAs, respectively. However, the bioconversion of ALA to EPA and DHA is low, suggesting the importance of dietary intake of these nutrients to achieve optimal status.[20] Over the past several decades, potential changes in the Western diet have included an increase in n-6 PUFA intake from increased consumption of vegetable oils and other food sources[58,59] along with potential concomitant decrease in n-3 PFUA intake from decreased oily fish intake with a subsequent relevant increase in the n-6:n3 fatty acid ratio.[50,59]

Prenatal Polyunsaturated Acids and Child Asthma and Allergy Outcomes

Multiple longitudinal pregnancy cohorts have investigated associations between prenatal PUFAs and child asthma and allergy outcomes with inconsistent results.[11,24,30] Findings from observational studies and clinical trials have reported associations with higher maternal n-3 prenatal intake or biomarker status or supplementation with decreased wheeze/asthma outcomes in children in some but not all investigations.[11,32,37,41,60–65] Although results have been inconsistent, several studies and systematic reviews provide some support that higher prenatal n-3 PUFAs are decreased wheeze/asthma and atopic disease.[32,34,36,37,55,60,65,66] In a randomized controlled trial, Bisgaard and colleagues found that maternal prenatal fish oil supplementation was associated with decreased child wheeze and asthma in children up to 5 years of age, with the largest effects in women with lower n-3 PUFA levels at randomization.[31] Studies have also investigated the association between prenatal n-6 PUFA intake and the n6:n3 PUFA ratio and child asthma and allergic outcomes. Investigations have found that higher n-6 PUFA intake was associated with eczema[67] and asthma[68] and a higher n-6:n-3 PUFA was associated with allergic rhinitis[69] in some but not all studies.[63,66] In addition, associations between n-6 PUFAs assessed using biomarker data have detected associations between higher n-6 PUFA or the n6:n3 ratio and increased child asthma and atopic disease outcomes.[11,30,66] Taken together, environmental changes that impact the abundance and infrastructure of the ecosystem on n-3 PUFAs or alters the n-6:n3 PUFA ratio have potential implications regarding prenatal influences of child asthma and allergy.

Impact of Climate Change on the Distribution and Abundance of Omega-3 and Omega-6 Fatty Acids

Anthropogenic global climate change is associated with increase in greenhouse gases emission contributing to the warming of the earth's climate at an accelerated pace than would occur naturally.[20,70] Associated changes include decreases in stratospheric ozone layer with subsequent increase in ultraviolet-B irradiation, increase in temperature in the earth's aquatic ecosystems, and ocean acidification.[19,20,70] These changes have the potential to impact the future abundance and composition of LC-PUFAs which are sensitive to climate-related environmental changes. Long-chain n-3 PUFAs are fatty acids found primarily in animal-based foods, with fish oil being the major source of EPA and DHA in the human diet. Marine phytoplankton are the main producers of n-3 fatty acids in the food web[71–74] and can be obtained in the human diet through multiple levels.[20] Phytoplankton are sensitive to the effects of environmental and climate change, including increasing global temperature, ocean surface temperature, carbon dioxide (CO_2), and ocean acidification.[15,19] Phytoplankton are also particularly sensitive to effects of UVB radiation with negative effects on photosynthesis and DNA.[20] In the context of modeling, the impact of global climate change on the fatty acid content of phytoplankton in aquatic systems, Hixson and Arts observed that increasing water temperature was generally associated with decreases in EPA and DHA and increases in LA and AA production.[21] Tan and colleagues did an extensive review of investigations that included laboratory, field, and model simulations that taken together highlight how climate change may impact n-3 LC PUFA abundance.[19] Potential effects include decreasing the primary producers of n-3 fatty acids, alteration of the community structure of phytoplankton, negatively impacting the quality and quantity of LC-PUFAs, and decreased n-3 PUFAs and n-3/n-6 ratio.[19,20]

Prenatal Oxidative Stress, Antioxidants, and Child Asthma

Systemic OS is a potential mediator of asthma and atopic disease.[75] In vitro data support that ROS exposure can upregulate Th2 cytokine response.[76] This process is inhibited with antioxidant exposure, suggesting the ROS/antioxidant balance is important for immune response and asthma.[76] One process of OS is lipid peroxidation resulting from oxidants interacting with carbon–carbon double bond containing lipids, such as PUFAs, primarily AA[77] and products of lipid peroxidation include F_2-isoprostanes (F_2-IsoPs). F_2-IsoPs influence multiple cellular processes in the lung and have been implicated in asthma such that prolonged elevated exposure may influence airway remodeling or function.[78–81] Individuals with asthma, including children in stable condition,[82,83] have increased F_2-IsoPs in exhaled breath condensate,[84–88] urine,[89] and plasma[90] compared with individuals without asthma. Pregnancy is associated with enhanced susceptibility to OS,[78] which contributes to pregnancy-associated illnesses including preeclampsia.[56,91–94] In overlapping research, pregnancy-associated illnesses, including diabetes mellitus and preeclampsia, have been linked with child wheeze.[78,94–96] Altered fetal antioxidant/oxidant balance may result in oxidative injury of the developing lung or immune system.[97–99] The developing fetus has limited antioxidant protection and may experience detrimental developmental effects when OS defenses are overwhelmed.[100,101]

Prenatal dietary antioxidants are important for lung growth and immune development.[102] For example, vitamin E is a micronutrient that includes several isomers including alpha-and gamma-tocopherol. Alpha-tocopherol is particularly relevant as the primary antioxidant to counteract the effects of lipid peroxyl radicals.[78] Higher prenatal vitamin E intake is associated with decreased early life wheeze[28,29,103] and decreased current wheeze and doctor diagnosed asthma at 5 years.[27] Increased plasma alpha-tocopherol levels are associated with decreased wheeze and correlated with higher post-bronchodilator FEV1 at age 5 years after adjusting for the child's intakes.[27] Alpha-tocopherol has been associated with fetal somatic growth[104,105] that, in turn, is positively associated with lung function and inversely associated with childhood wheeze/asthma.[104] Research suggests the need for studying effects of higher alpha-tocopherol and its anti-inflammatory effects in the setting of low levels of the proinflammatory gamma-tocopherol.[106] Furthermore, investigations between prenatal OS, measured by a mix of F_2-isoprostanes with 8-iso-prostaglandin $F_{2\alpha}$[107,108] as the predominant isomer, and childhood respiratory outcomes in mother–child dyads found that associations between prenatal F_2-IsoPs and child wheeze/asthma in some but not all subpopulations.[109]

Climate Change and Vegetable Crop Nutritional Quality

Climate change and its manifestations including extreme temperatures, changes in relative humidity, flooding, wild fires, drought, and sea-level rise affect agricultural ecosystems through adverse impacts on abiotic processes including soil water deficits and soil salinity.[110] Rising CO_2 levels, droughts and soil water deficits, and salinity influence the availability and nutritional quality of food sources including vegetable crop antioxidant properties,[25,26,111] therefore alternations in crop quality or yield may have health implications. Beans and lentils are edible seeds of legumes and typically are rich sources of vegetable protein and micronutrients with antioxidant properties that are important contributors to a high-quality diet.[112,113] Bansal and colleagues[25] found that water limitation in an experimental setting was associated with reduced lentil seed yield and weight, decreases in nutrients such as protein, iron, and zinc, as well as a measure of antioxidant activity.[25] In addition, this work detected genotypes that may be more resistant to specific stressors, such as water limitation or drought that provide insights regarding agricultural methods that may be used to address effects of climate change. Elevated CO_2 levels may also adversely affect nutrient quality.[26] In a meta-analysis of experimental investigations, Myers and colleagues reported that elevated CO_2 levels were associated with decreased concentration of iron, zinc, and protein in the edible portion of several crops including grains (wheat, rice) and legumes (field peas) when compared with crops grown at ambient CO_2 levels.[26] Emerging studies have highlighted the importance of considering agricultural interventions may be used to increase the antioxidant or nutritional quality of crops.[111,114]

In summary, asthma and related childhood allergic disorders are complex conditions and the environmental effects of uncurbed climate change will have important implications for disease incidence and morbidity. In addition to adverse effects on child respiratory and allergy conditions through climate-related changes in ambient environmental toxicants and allergens, it will be important to consider climate effects on dietary nutritional quality, including nutrients known to influence disease expression such as PUFAs and dietary antioxidants.

CLINICS CARE POINTS

- Clinicians should have insight into the effects of climate change and potential impact on asthma and allergic disorders.
- In addition to influence on ambient environmental triggers and allergens, climate change also influences ecologic systems that may affect the quality and availability of nutrients.
- As associations between prenatal polyunsaturated fatty acids and antioxidants are further delineated, the impact of climate change may be important in understanding trends of asthma and allergic disease and informing prevention efforts.

DISCLOSURE

Dr Carroll receives grant funding from the National Institutes of Health.

REFERENCES

1. Serebrisky D, Wiznia A. Pediatric Asthma: A Global Epidemic. Ann Glob Health 2019;85(1). https://doi.org/10.5334/aogh.2416.

2. Stern J, Pier J, Litonjua AA. Asthma epidemiology and risk factors. Semin Immunopathol 2020;42(1):5–15.
3. García-Marcos L, Asher MI, Pearce N, et al. The burden of asthma, hay fever and eczema in children in 25 countries: GAN Phase I study. Eur Respir J 2022;60(3). https://doi.org/10.1183/13993003.02866-2021.
4. Singh AB, Kumar P. Climate change and allergic diseases: An overview. Front Allergy 2022;3:964987.
5. Gokhale M, Hattori T, Evitt L, et al. Burden of asthma exacerbations and health care utilization in pediatric patients with asthma in the US and England. Immun Inflamm Dis 2020;8(2):236–45.
6. Perry R, Braileanu G, Palmer T, et al. The Economic Burden of Pediatric Asthma in the United States: Literature Review of Current Evidence. Pharmacoeconomics 2019;37(2):155–67.
7. Agrawal S, Iqbal S, Patel SJ, et al. Quality of life in at-risk school-aged children with asthma. J Asthma 2021;58(12):1680–8.
8. Fazel N, Kundi M, Jensen-Jarolim E, et al. Quality of life and asthma control in pregnant women with asthma. BMC Pulm Med 2021;21(1):415.
9. Kim KW, Ober C. Lessons Learned From GWAS of Asthma. Allergy Asthma Immunol Res 2019;11(2):170–87.
10. Beerweiler CC, Masanetz RK, Schaub B. Asthma and allergic diseases: Cross talk of immune system and environmental factors. Eur J Immunol 2023;53(6): e2249981.
11. Rosa MJ, Hartman TJ, Adgent M, et al. Prenatal polyunsaturated fatty acids and child asthma: Effect modification by maternal asthma and child sex. J Allergy Clin Immunol 2020;145(3):800–807 e4.
12. Lee A, Mathilda Chiu YH, Rosa MJ, et al. Prenatal and postnatal stress and asthma in children: Temporal- and sex-specific associations. J Allergy Clin Immunol 2016;138(3):740–7, e3. Not in File.
13. Carroll KN, Hartert TV. The impact of respiratory viral infection on wheezing illnesses and asthma exacerbations. ImmunolAllergy ClinNorth Am 2008;28(3): 539–61, viii. Not in File.
14. Makrufardi F, Manullang A, Rusmawatiningtyas D, et al. Extreme weather and asthma: a systematic review and meta-analysis. Eur Respir Rev 2023;32(168). https://doi.org/10.1183/16000617.0019-2023.
15. Wright RJ. Influences of climate change on childhood asthma and allergy risk. Lancet Child Adolesc Health 2020;4(12):859–60.
16. Kline O, Prunicki M. Climate change impacts on children's respiratory health. Curr Opin Pediatr 2023;35(3):350–5.
17. D'Amato G, D'Amato M. Climate change, air pollution, pollen allergy and extreme atmospheric events. Curr Opin Pediatr 2023;35(3):356–61.
18. Deng S, Han A, Jin S, et al. Effect of extreme temperatures on asthma hospital visits: Modification by event characteristics and healthy behaviors. Environ Res 2023;226:115679.
19. Tan K, Zhang H, Zheng H. Climate change and n-3 LC-PUFA availability. Prog Lipid Res 2022;86:101161.
20. Kang JX. Omega-3: a link between global climate change and human health. Biotechnol Adv 2011;29(4):388–90.
21. Hixson SM, Arts MT. Climate warming is predicted to reduce omega-3, long-chain, polyunsaturated fatty acid production in phytoplankton. Glob Chang Biol 2016;22(8):2744–55.

22. Noakes PS, Vlachava M, Kremmyda LS, et al. Increased intake of oily fish in pregnancy: effects on neonatal immune responses and on clinical outcomes in infants at 6 mo. Am J Clin Nutr 2012;95(2):395–404.

23. McEvoy CT, Schilling D, Clay N, et al. Vitamin C supplementation for pregnant smoking women and pulmonary function in their newborn infants: a randomized clinical trial. JAMA 2014;311(20):2074–82. Not in File.

24. Miles EA, Childs CE, Calder PC. Long-Chain Polyunsaturated Fatty Acids (LCPUFAs) and the Developing Immune System: A Narrative Review. Nutrients 2021;13(1). https://doi.org/10.3390/nu13010247.

25. Bansal R, Bana RS, Dikshit HK, et al. Seed nutritional quality in lentil (Lens culinaris) under different moisture regimes. Front Nutr 2023;10:1141040.

26. Myers SS, Zanobetti A, Kloog I, et al. Increasing CO_2 threatens human nutrition. Nature 2014;510(7503):139–42.

27. Devereux G, Turner SW, Craig LC, et al. Low maternal vitamin E intake during pregnancy is associated with asthma in 5-year-old children. Am J Respir Crit Care Med 2006;174(5):499–507.

28. Miyake Y, Sasaki S, Tanaka K, et al. Consumption of vegetables, fruit, and antioxidants during pregnancy and wheeze and eczema in infants. Allergy 2010; 65(6):758–65.

29. Martindale S, McNeill G, Devereux G, et al. Antioxidant intake in pregnancy in relation to wheeze and eczema in the first two years of life. Am J Respir Crit Care Med 2005;171(2):121–8. Not in File.

30. Gardner KG, Gebretsadik T, Hartman TJ, et al. Prenatal Omega-3 and Omega-6 Polyunsaturated Fatty Acids and Childhood Atopic Dermatitis. J Allergy Clin Immunol Pract 2019. https://doi.org/10.1016/j.jaip.2019.09.031.

31. Bisgaard H, Stokholm J, Chawes BL, et al. Fish Oil-Derived Fatty Acids in Pregnancy and Wheeze and Asthma in Offspring. N Engl J Med 2016;375(26): 2530–9.

32. Jia Y, Huang Y, Wang H, et al. A dose-response meta-analysis of the association between the maternal omega-3 long-chain polyunsaturated fatty acids supplement and risk of asthma/wheeze in offspring. BMC Pediatr 2022;22(1):422.

33. Chiu YM, Carroll KN, Coull BA, et al. Prenatal Fine Particulate Matter, Maternal Micronutrient Antioxidant Intake, and Early Childhood Repeated Wheeze: Effect Modification by Race/Ethnicity and Sex. Antioxidants 2022;11(2). https://doi.org/10.3390/antiox11020366.

34. Dotterud CK, Storro O, Simpson MR, et al. The impact of pre- and postnatal exposures on allergy related diseases in childhood: a controlled multicentre intervention study in primary health care. BMC Publ Health 2013;13:123. Not in File.

35. Cook-Mills J, Gebretsadik T, Abdala-Valencia H, et al. Interaction of vitamin E isoforms on asthma and allergic airway disease. Thorax. Oct 2016;71(10): 954–6.

36. Jia Y, Huang Y, Wang H, et al. Effect of Prenatal Omega-3 Polyunsaturated Fatty Acid Supplementation on Childhood Eczema: A Systematic Review and Meta-Analysis. Int Arch Allergy Immunol 2023;184(1):21–32.

37. Kachroo P, Kelly RS, Mirzakhani H, et al. Fish oil supplementation during pregnancy is protective against asthma/wheeze in offspring. J Allergy Clin Immunol Pract 2020;8(1):388–91.e2.

38. Calder PC. n-3 polyunsaturated fatty acids, inflammation, and inflammatory diseases. Am J Clin Nutr 2006;83(6 Suppl):1505S–19S.

39. Calder PC, Kremmyda LS, Vlachava M, et al. Is there a role for fatty acids in early life programming of the immune system? Proc Nutr Soc 2010 2010; 69(3):373–80.
40. Prescott SL, Dunstan JA. Prenatal fatty acid status and immune development: the pathways and the evidence. Lipids 2007;42(9):801–10. Not in File.
41. Sordillo JE, Rifas-Shiman SL, Switkowski K, et al. Prenatal oxidative balance and risk of asthma and allergic disease in adolescence. J Allergy Clin Immunol 2019;144(6):1534–41.e5.
42. Traina G, Bolzacchini E, Bonini M, et al. Role of air pollutants mediated oxidative stress in respiratory diseases. Pediatr Allergy Immunol 2022;33(Suppl 27): 38–40.
43. Pate CA, Zahran HS, Qin X, et al. Asthma Surveillance - United States, 2006-2018. MMWR Surveill Summ 2021;70(5):1–32.
44. Miller RL, Schuh H, Chandran A, et al. Incidence rates of childhood asthma with recurrent exacerbations in the US Environmental influences on Child Health Outcomes (ECHO) program. J Allergy Clin Immunol 2023;152(1):84–93.
45. Krauss-Etschmann S, Hartl D, Rzehak P, et al. Decreased cord blood IL-4, IL-13, and CCR4 and increased TGF-beta levels after fish oil supplementation of pregnant women. J Allergy Clin Immunol 2008;121(2):464–70. Not in File.
46. Dunstan JA, Mori TA, Barden A, et al. Fish oil supplementation in pregnancy modifies neonatal allergen-specific immune responses and clinical outcomes in infants at high risk of atopy: a randomized, controlled trial. J Allergy Clin Immunol 2003;112(6):1178–84. Not in File.
47. Indrio F, Martini S, Francavilla R, et al. Epigenetic Matters: The Link between Early Nutrition, Microbiome, and Long-term Health Development. Front Pediatr 2017;5:178.
48. Acevedo N, Alashkar Alhamwe B, Caraballo L, et al. Perinatal and Early-Life Nutrition, Epigenetics, and Allergy. Nutrients 2021;13(3). https://doi.org/10.3390/nu13030724.
49. Wiktorowska-Owczarek A, Berezińska M, Nowak JZ. PUFAs: Structures, Metabolism and Functions. Adv Clin Exp Med 2015;24(6):931–41.
50. Mariamenatu AH, Abdu EM. Overconsumption of Omega-6 Polyunsaturated Fatty Acids (PUFAs) versus Deficiency of Omega-3 PUFAs in Modern-Day Diets: The Disturbing Factor for Their "Balanced Antagonistic Metabolic Functions" in the Human Body. Journal of Lipids 2021;2021:8848161.
51. Calder PC. Polyunsaturated fatty acids and cytokine profiles: a clue to the changing prevalence of atopy? Clin Exp Allergy 2003;33(4):412–5.
52. Calder PC. N-3 polyunsaturated fatty acids and inflammation: from molecular biology to the clinic. Lipids 2003;38(4):343–52.
53. Pham MN, Bunyavanich S. Prenatal Diet and the Development of Childhood Allergic Diseases: Food for Thought. Curr Allergy Asthma Rep 2018;18(11):58.
54. Montes R, Chisaguano AM, Castellote AI, et al. Fatty-acid composition of maternal and umbilical cord plasma and early childhood atopic eczema in a Spanish cohort. European Journal Of Clinical Nutrition 2013;67(6):658–63.
55. Klemens CM, Berman DR, Mozurkewich EL. The effect of perinatal omega-3 fatty acid supplementation on inflammatory markers and allergic diseases: a systematic review. BJOG 2011;118(8):916–25. Not in File.
56. Jones ML, Mark PJ, Mori TA, et al. Maternal dietary omega-3 fatty acid supplementation reduces placental oxidative stress and increases fetal and placental growth in the rat. Biol Reprod 2013;88(2):37. Not in File.

57. Kremmyda LS, Vlachava M, Noakes PS, et al. Atopy risk in infants and children in relation to early exposure to fish, oily fish, or long-chain omega-3 fatty acids: a systematic review. Clin RevAllergy Immunol 2011;41(1):36–66. Not in File.

58. Blasbalg TL, Hibbeln JR, Ramsden CE, et al. Changes in consumption of omega-3 and omega-6 fatty acids in the United States during the 20th century. Am J Clin Nutr 2011;93(5):950–62.

59. Black PN, Sharpe S. Dietary fat and asthma: is there a connection? Eur Respir J 1997;10(1):6–12.

60. Pike KC, Calder PC, Inskip HM, et al. Maternal plasma phosphatidylcholine fatty acids and atopy and wheeze in the offspring at age of 6 years. Clin Dev Immunol 2012;2012:474613. Not in File.

61. Miyake Y, Sasaki S, Tanaka K, et al. Maternal fat consumption during pregnancy and risk of wheeze and eczema in Japanese infants aged 16-24 months: the Osaka Maternal and Child Health Study. Thorax 2009;64(9):815–21. Not in File.

62. Stratakis N, Conti DV, Borras E, et al. Association of Fish Consumption and Mercury Exposure During Pregnancy With Metabolic Health and Inflammatory Biomarkers in Children. JAMA Network Open 2020;3(3):e201007.

63. Rucci E, den Dekker HT, de Jongste JC, et al. Maternal fatty acid levels during pregnancy, childhood lung function and atopic diseases. The Generation R Study. Clin Exp Allergy 2016;46(3):461–71.

64. Olsen SF, Osterdal ML, Salvig JD, et al. Fish oil intake compared with olive oil intake in late pregnancy and asthma in the offspring: 16 y of registry-based follow-up from a randomized controlled trial. Am J Clin Nutr 2008;88(1): 167–75. Not in File.

65. Furuhjelm C, Warstedt K, Larsson J, et al. Fish oil supplementation in pregnancy and lactation may decrease the risk of infant allergy. Acta Paediatr 2009;98(9): 1461–7.

66. Notenboom ML, Mommers M, Jansen EH, et al. Maternal fatty acid status in pregnancy and childhood atopic manifestations: KOALA Birth Cohort Study. Clin ExpAllergy 2011;41(3):407–16. Not in File.

67. Miyake Y, Sasaki S, Tanaka K, et al. Maternal B vitamin intake during pregnancy and wheeze and eczema in Japanese infants aged 16-24 months: The Osaka Maternal and Child Health Study. Pediatr Allergy Immunol 2010. ;Not in File.

68. Flom JD, Chiu YM, Cowell W, et al. Maternal active asthma in pregnancy influences associations between polyunsaturated fatty acid intake and child asthma. Ann Allergy Asthma Immunol 2021;127(5):553–61.

69. Nwaru BI, Erkkola M, Lumia M, et al. Maternal intake of fatty acids during pregnancy and allergies in the offspring. BrJNutr 2012;108(4):720–32. Not in File.

70. Poole JA, Barnes CS, Demain JG, et al. Impact of weather and climate change with indoor and outdoor air quality in asthma: A Work Group Report of the AAAAI Environmental Exposure and Respiratory Health Committee. J Allergy Clin Immunol 2019;143(5):1702–10.

71. Li-Beisson Y, Thelen JJ, Fedosejevs E, et al. The lipid biochemistry of eukaryotic algae. Prog Lipid Res 2019;74:31–68.

72. Zulu NN, Zienkiewicz K, Vollheyde K, et al. Current trends to comprehend lipid metabolism in diatoms. Prog Lipid Res 2018;70:1–16.

73. Mühlroth A, Li K, Røkke G, et al. Pathways of lipid metabolism in marine algae, co-expression network, bottlenecks and candidate genes for enhanced production of EPA and DHA in species of Chromista. Mar Drugs 2013;11(11):4662–97.

74. Monroig Ó, Shu-Chien AC, Kabeya N, et al. Desaturases and elongases involved in long-chain polyunsaturated fatty acid biosynthesis in aquatic animals: From genes to functions. Prog Lipid Res 2022;86:101157.

75. Bowler RP, Crapo JD. Oxidative stress in allergic respiratory diseases. J Allergy Clin Immunol 2002;110(3):349–56.

76. King MR, Ismail AS, Davis LS, et al. Oxidative stress promotes polarization of human T cell differentiation toward a T helper 2 phenotype. J Immunol 2006; 176(5):2765–72.

77. Ayala A, Munoz MF, Arguelles S. Lipid peroxidation: production, metabolism, and signaling mechanisms of malondialdehyde and 4-hydroxy-2-nonenal. Oxidative Medicine And Cellular Longevity 2014;360438. https://doi.org/10.1155/2014/360438.

78. Burton GJ, Jauniaux E. Oxidative stress. Best Pract Res Clin Obstet Gynaecol 2011;25(3):287–99.

79. Morrow JD, Hill KE, Burk RF, et al. A series of prostaglandin F2-like compounds are produced in vivo in humans by a non-cyclooxygenase, free radical-catalyzed mechanism. Proc Natl Acad Sci U S A. Dec 1990;87(23):9383–7.

80. Roberts LJ 2nd, Milne GL. Isoprostanes. J Lipid Res 2009;50(Suppl):S219–23. https://doi.org/10.1194/jlr.R800037-JLR200.

81. Voynow JA, Kummarapurugu A. Isoprostanes and asthma. Biochimica et biophysica acta 2011;1810(11):1091–5.

82. Baraldi E, Ghiro L, Piovan V, et al. Increased exhaled 8-isoprostane in childhood asthma. Chest 2003;124(1):25–31.

83. Zanconato S, Carraro S, Corradi M, et al. Leukotrienes and 8-isoprostane in exhaled breath condensate of children with stable and unstable asthma. J Allergy Clin Immunol. Feb 2004;113(2):257–63.

84. Montuschi P, Corradi M, Ciabattoni G, et al. Increased 8-isoprostane, a marker of oxidative stress, in exhaled condensate of asthma patients. Am J Respir Crit Care Med 1999;160(1):216–20.

85. Baraldi E, Carraro S, Alinovi R, et al. Cysteinyl leukotrienes and 8-isoprostane in exhaled breath condensate of children with asthma exacerbations. Thorax 2003;58(6):505–9.

86. Shahid SK, Kharitonov SA, Wilson NM, et al. Exhaled 8-isoprostane in childhood asthma. Respir Res 2005;6:79.

87. Wedes SH, Khatri SB, Zhang R, et al. Noninvasive markers of airway inflammation in asthma. Clinical And Translational Science 2009;2(2):112–7.

88. Barreto M, Villa MP, Olita C, et al. 8-Isoprostane in exhaled breath condensate and exercise-induced bronchoconstriction in asthmatic children and adolescents. Chest 2009;135(1):66–73.

89. Dworski R, Roberts LJ 2nd, Murray JJ, et al. Assessment of oxidant stress in allergic asthma by measurement of the major urinary metabolite of F2-isoprostane, 15-F2t-IsoP (8-iso-PGF2alpha). Clin Exp Allergy 2001;31(3): 387–90.

90. Wood LG, Fitzgerald DA, Gibson PG, et al. Lipid peroxidation as determined by plasma isoprostanes is related to disease severity in mild asthma. Lipids 2000; 35(9):967–74.

91. Bilodeau JF, Qin Wei S, Larose J, et al. Plasma F2-isoprostane class VI isomers at 12-18 weeks of pregnancy are associated with later occurrence of pre-eclampsia. Free Radical Biol Med 2015;85:282–7.

92. Myatt L, Cui X. Oxidative stress in the placenta. Histochem Cell Biol 2004; 122(4):369–82.

93. Redman CW, Sargent IL. Placental stress and pre-eclampsia: a revised view. Placenta 2009;30(Suppl A):S38–42.

94. Adgent MA, Gebretsadik T, Reedus J, et al. Gestational diabetes and childhood asthma in a racially diverse US pregnancy cohort. Pediatr Allergy Immunol 2021;32(6):1190–6.

95. Rusconi F, Galassi C, Forastiere F, et al. Maternal complications and procedures in pregnancy and at birth and wheezing phenotypes in children. Am J Respir Crit Care Med 2007;175(1):16–21.

96. De Luca G, Olivieri F, Melotti G, et al. Fetal and early postnatal life roots of asthma. J Matern Fetal Neonatal Med 2010;23(Suppl 3):80–3.

97. Weinberger B, Nisar S, Anwar M, et al. Lipid peroxidation in cord blood and neonatal outcome. Pediatr Int 2006;48(5):479–83.

98. Belik J, Gonzalez-Luis GE, Perez-Vizcaino F, et al. Isoprostanes in fetal and neonatal health and disease. Free Radical Biol Med 2010;48(2):177–88.

99. Mestan K, Matoba N, Arguelles L, et al. Cord blood 8-isoprostane in the preterm infant. Early Hum Dev 2012;88(8):683–9.

100. Suh DI, Chang HY, Lee E, et al. Prenatal Maternal Distress and Allergic Diseases in Offspring: Review of Evidence and Possible Pathways. Allergy Asthma Immunol Res 2017;9(3):200–11.

101. de Wijs-Meijler DP, Duncker DJ, Tibboel D, et al. Oxidative injury of the pulmonary circulation in the perinatal period: Short- and long-term consequences for the human cardiopulmonary system. Pulm Circ 2017;7(1):55–66.

102. Nurmatov U, Devereux G, Sheikh A. Nutrients and foods for the primary prevention of asthma and allergy: systematic review and meta-analysis. J Allergy Clin Immunol 2011;127(3):724–33, e1-30. Not in File.

103. Beckhaus AA, Garcia-Marcos L, Forno E, et al. Maternal nutrition during pregnancy and risk of asthma, wheeze, and atopic diseases during childhood: a systematic review and meta-analysis. Allergy 2015;70(12):1588–604.

104. Turner SW, Campbell D, Smith N, et al. Associations between fetal size, maternal {alpha}-tocopherol and childhood asthma. Thorax 2010;65(5):391–7. Not in File.

105. Scholl TO, Chen X, Sims M, et al. Vitamin C: maternal concentrations are associated with fetal growth. AmJClinNutr 2006;84(6):1442–8. Not in File.

106. Cook-Mills JM, bdala-Valencia H, Hartert T. Two faces of vitamin e in the lung. Am J Respir Crit Care Med 2013;188(3):279–84. Not in File.

107. Tylavsky FA, Han L, Sims Taylor LM, et al. Oxidative Balance Score during Pregnancy Is Associated with Oxidative Stress in the CANDLE Study. Nutrients 2022; 14(11). https://doi.org/10.3390/nu14112327.

108. Chung CP, Schmidt D, Stein CM, et al. Increased oxidative stress in patients with depression and its relationship to treatment. Psychiatr Res 2013;206(2–3): 213–6.

109. Adgent MA, Gebretsadik T, Elaiho CR, et al. The association between prenatal F(2)-isoprostanes and child wheeze/asthma and modification by maternal race. Free Radical Biol Med 2022;189:85–90.

110. Mukhopadhyay R, Sarkar B, Jat HS, et al. Soil salinity under climate change: Challenges for sustainable agriculture and food security. J Environ Manage 2021;280:111736.

111. Abd El Mageed TA, Semida W, Hemida KA, et al. Glutathione-mediated changes in productivity, photosynthetic efficiency, osmolytes, and antioxidant capacity of common beans (Phaseolus vulgaris) grown under water deficit. PeerJ 2023;11:e15343.

112. Ganesan K, Xu B. Polyphenol-Rich Lentils and Their Health Promoting Effects. Int J Mol Sci 2017;18(11). https://doi.org/10.3390/ijms18112390.
113. Vassilopoulou E, Guibas GV, Papadopoulos NG. Mediterranean-Type Diets as a Protective Factor for Asthma and Atopy. Nutrients 2022;14(9). https://doi.org/10.3390/nu14091825.
114. Halawani RF, AbdElgawad H, Aloufi FA, et al. Synergistic effect of carbon nanoparticles with mild salinity for improving chemical composition and antioxidant activities of radish sprouts. Front Plant Sci 2023;14:1158031.

Methods to Advance Climate Science in Respiratory Health

Satellite-Based Environmental Modeling for Temperature Exposure Assessment in Epidemiological Studies

Itai Kloog, PhD[a,b,c,1], Xueying Zhang, PhD[a,c,d,1],*

KEYWORDS

- Environmental modeling • Air temperature • Ambient temperature
- Environmental epidemiology • Public health • Remote sensing

KEY POINTS

- Earth observation data allow the advancement of exposure assessment in temperature modeling for climate science.
- Spatiotemporally resolved air temperature at the residence resolution can reduce exposure bias in estimated health effects and improve our understanding of human adaptation to temperature.
- Extremes in high or low temperature are associated with adverse respiratory outcomes.
- Temperature can enhance the impacts of ambient air pollution on respiratory outcomes.

BACKGROUND

Scientific consensus strongly supports the scenario that greenhouse gas emissions and air pollution generated by human activity are changing the global climate.[1] This change in climate will lead to warmer air temperature and more extreme weather events with greater heat stress, which in turn are associated with increased morbidity

a Department of Environmental Medicine and Public Health, Icahn School of Medicine at Mount Sinai, New York, NY, USA; b Department of Geography and Environmental Development, Ben-Gurion University, Beer Sheva, Israel; c Institute for Exposomic Research, Icahn School of Medicine at Mount Sinai, New York, NY, USA; d Department of Pediatrics, The Kravis Children's Hospital, Icahn School of Medicine at Mount Sinai, New York, NY, USA
1 Equal co-author status, both authors contributed equally to this work.
* Corresponding author. Department of Environmental Medicine and Public Health, Icahn School of Medicine at Mount Sinai, New York, NY 10029.
E-mail address: xueying.zhang@mssm.edu

Immunol Allergy Clin N Am 44 (2024) 97–107
https://doi.org/10.1016/j.iac.2023.07.002
0889-8561/24/© 2023 Elsevier Inc. All rights reserved.

and mortality. The global average air temperatures are predicted to increase between 1.4°C and 4.4°C by the year 2100 with respect to the temperature from 1850 to 1900.[2] The ongoing climate change is attributed to the impacts of population growth and increased consumption.[3] Although climate change is widely accepted by the scientific community and many governments,[4] the extent of its impacts are still unclear. Understanding the direct effects of climate change on human health will inform more refined policies to protect the health of communities and populations across the globe.

Epidemiological studies have described a substantial increase in morbidity and mortality in conjunction with heat episodes,[5] of which the 2003 heat wave in Europe is a well-known example.[6] Heat stress may be additionally exacerbated by the urban heat island (UHI), which is a localized anthropogenic climate modification in the urban atmosphere, especially in the urban canopy layer where most human activity occurs[7] and greater respiratory morbidity is also documented. Variable temperatures (such as low, high, and extreme exposures) have been associated with increased morbidity and mortality across varied regions and climates.[8–11] The elderly[12] and children,[13] especially the old and infants, are particularly at risk for a variety of conditions including cardiovascular,[14] cerebrovascular,[12] and respiratory diseases.[12] Heat effects are mostly short term (lag 0–3 days) whereas cold effects lag by up to 30 days.[12] Temperature also affects health through its role in the prevalence and distribution of vector-borne and infectious diseases[15] and its interaction with air pollution.[16]

This review provides an overview of the current state of the art methods for estimating air temperature from earth observing satellite data and its application in environmental health studies. The first sections of the review "*Exposure misclassification*," "*Traditional modeling of air pollution*," "*Hybrid modeling, incorporating earth observation data into temperature exposure modeling*," and "*Estimating air temperature from land surface temperature*" describe how land surface temperature (LST) is used to derive air temperature (Ta) for health studies. "*Satellite-derived air temperature and respiratory outcomes in environmental health studies*" and "*Air temperature enhanced the effects of air pollution on respiratory outcomes*" summarize recent epidemiological studies using these generated Ta predictions for investigating adverse health outcomes focusing on respiratory outcomes related to temperature exposures.

EXPOSURE MISCLASSIFICATION

Until recent years, environmental health studies on the association between temperature and human health have traditionally estimated exposures for an entire city or across countries based on the air temperature (also known as ambient temperature or near-surface temperature) measured at one or a few monitoring stations that is available close to the residence. Although most of these studies focus on urban areas, where the bulk of the population is found, even the nearest station could be several kilometers away. The study populations might even be exposed to a different microclimate due to fine scale intra-urban gradients, potentially biasing the health effect risk estimates due to exposure measurement error (also known as exposure bias or exposure misclassification, ie, assigning inaccurate exposure to each study participant)[17] which may result in a downward bias in estimated health effects. Thus, development of better exposure assessment methods were critical to handle available health outcome datasets, which are often misaligned in both time and space.

TRADITIONAL MODELING OF TEMPERATURE

To address this issue of exposure misclassification, researchers have explored a multitude of methods to produce spatially continuous high-resolution temperature surfaces for use in the fields of public health, meteorology, climatology, hydrology, and ecology. Techniques have varied in complexity from simple interpolations to advanced downscaling models.[18] Many groups in the last decade have explored the use of advanced statistics and geospatial models such as advance linear mixed models, complex space–time interpolations, and land use regression methods.[19–21] These models while improving upon early efforts for spatial temperature variations are still limited in their temporal extent and are inadequate for capturing daily and intra-daily temperature variations.

HYBRID MODELING: INCORPORATING EARTH OBSERVATION DATA INTO TEMPERATURE EXPOSURE MODELING

Access to large administrative databases (eg, NASA satellite data) obtained via satellite remote sensing make it possible to efficiently collect and use climate and weather-related data to facilitate place-based respiratory health research. Earth observation data (from orbiting satellites) provide us with land skin temperature or LST data, which are derived from measured thermal radiation using Planck's law and adjusting for atmospheric effects and surface emissivity.[22] LST is used as a proxy for air temperature, and thus multiple groups have explored the use of LST to model ground level air temperature (Ta). The broad spatial coverage enabled by these satellites allows us to expand exposure data far beyond the range of conventional ground monitoring networks to penetrate rural and suburban areas. This greatly enhances our ability to estimate subject-specific exposures at place of residence and robustly reconstruct the spatial and temporal patterns of temperature exposure.[23–26]

One of the most widely used instruments for measuring LST is the moderate resolution imaging spectroradiometer (MODIS) carried by the Terra and Aqua satellites. MODIS has a 1 km spatial resolution LST product, and each satellite passes twice daily (equator crossing at 10:30 and 22:30 for Terra; 13:30 and 1:30 for Aqua). This results in a total of 4 MODIS measurements per day. Terra was launched in December 1999 and Aqua followed in May 2002. A validated higher-level (pre-calculated) twice daily 1 km LST product is freely available for each satellite.[27] The MODIS instrument's combination of a high temporal resolution (4 measures per day) and moderate spatial resolution (1 km) makes it well suited for many epidemiological studies. The NASA successor for MODIS, the Visible Infrared Imaging Radiometer Suite (VIIRS) is aboard the joint NASA/NOAA Suomi National Polar-orbiting Partnership (Suomi NPP) and NOAA-20 satellites. VIIRS, the successor to the MODIS platform, was launched in 2011 and collects visible and infrared imagery along with global observations of Earth's land, atmosphere, cryosphere, and ocean. It improves upon the spatial resolution of MODIS by providing data at 375 m resolution.[28]

ESTIMATING AIR TEMPERATURE FROM LAND SURFACE TEMPERATURE

Comparing to LST, T_a is a more precise measurement of the temperature that humans are exposed, and T_a is thereby used more often in public health research to investigate the adverse effects of ambient temperature. And as LST and T_a are closely related, studies developed modeling approaches to estimate T_a from LST data. The calibration and conversion between T_a from LST are complex.[29–31] Kloog and colleagues[23] were one of the first groups to develop a method using linear mixed models that explored the day-to-day variation in the LST–T_a relationship and allow for a robust calibration method. This multi-step geo-statistical approach also included a gap-filling stage that estimates T_a for day-locations where LST is unavailable based on information from nearby stations and predicted T_a at the location on days when LST is available.

The method has been later expanded to estimate daily T_a at 1 km resolution across the Northeastern United States (RMSE = 2.2 T_{mean}),[24] the Southeastern United States (RMSE = 1.4 T_{mean}),[25] France (RMSE = 1.7 T_{mean}),[26] and Israel (RMSE = 0.9 T_{mean}).[32]

Oyler and colleagues[33] presented a novel statistical framework for producing 800 m resolution gridded dataset of daily minimum and maximum temperature for an unprecedented period between 1948 and 2012 for the conterminous United States. They use weather station data and elevation-based predictors of temperature, while also implementing a unique spatiotemporal interpolation that incorporates remotely sensed 1 km LST temperature. The framework is able to capture several complex topo-climatic variations, including minimum temperature inversions, and represent spatial uncertainty in interpolated normal temperatures. They present excellent performance with mean absolute errors for annual normal minimum and maximum temperature of 0.78°C and 0.56°C, respectively.

New approaches in more recent studies have applied new machine learning methods to predict daily air temperature. Hough and colleagues[34] have modeled daily air temperature from 2000 to 2016 at a base resolution of 1 km^2 across continental France and at a 200 × 200 m^2 resolution across large urban areas. They predicted 3 Ta measures: minimum (T_{min}), mean (T_{mean}), and maximum (T_{max}). They calibrated daily Ta observations from weather stations with remotely sensed MODIS LST and other spatial predictors (eg, normalized difference vegetation index [NDVI], elevation) on a 1 km^2 grid. To increase the spatial resolution across large urban areas, they trained both random forest and extreme gradient boosting models to predict Ta predictions on a 200 × 200 m^2 grid. They used a generalized additive model (GAM) to ensemble the random forest and extreme gradient boosting predictions with weights that vary spatially and by the magnitude of the predicted residual. Model performance was excellent with RMSEs of 1.9°C, 1.3°C, and 1.8°C (T_{min}, T_{mean}, and T_{max}, respectively).

Jin and colleagues[35] applied a 3 stage ensemble model to estimate daily mean Ta from satellite-based LST over Sweden during 2001 to 2019 at a high spatial resolution of 1 × 1 km^2. The ensemble model incorporated 4 base models, including a GAM, a generalized additive mixed model, and 2 machine learning models (random forest and extreme gradient boosting), and allowed the weights for each model to vary over space, with the best-performing model for each grid cell assigned the highest weight. They included additional variables such as land cover type, NDVI, and elevation. Model performance was good and comparable to other machine-based exposure models with a RMSE of 1.38°C.

Flückiger and colleagues[36] applied a 2 stage approach using random forest to impute missing MODIS LST at a 1 × 1 km resolution and used this the gap-filled MODIS data to explain spatiotemporal variation in the measured ground-based air temperature data at a 100 × 100 m resolution across Switzerland. They used a range of predictor variables, including meteorological parameters, NDVI, impervious surface, and altitude. Their models managed to capture temporal and spatial variations in air temperature in Switzerland from 2003 to 2018 at a fine spatial resolution of 100 × 100 m. The models showed excellent performance with yearly RMSE ranging from 0.94°C to 1.86°C, respectively. They were also able to capture the UHI effect and some typical weather phenomena caused by Switzerland's complex topography.

Fig. 1 summarizes the general process common in many of the above-mentioned new modeling approaches. This starts with the geospatial collection of data (monitor data, satellite data, and all spatial and temporal variables). This is followed by a calibration stage, where the monitor Ta data are regressed against the satellite LST and all other geo-spatial predictors. Once robust model fits are achieved, the prediction stage

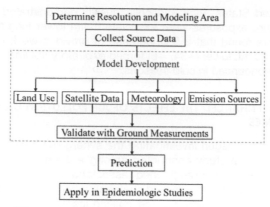

Fig. 1. General modeling process using earth observation data and hybrid modeling approaches.

takes place where new Ta data are generated based on the calibration model fits. All model stages are validated at each step. These final predictions are then distributed to collaborators and used in health outcome studies.

SATELLITE-DERIVED AIR TEMPERATURE AND RESPIRATORY DISEASES OUTCOMES IN ENVIRONMENTAL HEALTH STUDIES

The extreme weather and, in particular, the adverse health effects of ambient air temperature have been gaining both scientific and public interest in recent years. There have been multiple research articles using spatiotemporally resolved temperature data to examine the relationship between air temperature and adverse health outcomes. In this review, we focus on the adverse effect of temperature on respiratory disease outcomes. We divided the current literature into 2 groups based on how temperature was considered: studies using temperature as the main exposure and studies using temperature as an effect modifier.

A growing body of literature has shown that high-temperature exposure increases the risks of respiratory diseases outcomes, such as hospital admissions or incidence or exacerbation of respiratory diseases.[37–39] Studies in recent years leverage modeled temperature data that are increasingly spatiotemporally resolved to understand the adverse respiratory effects of ambient temperature exposure. Using gridded temperature data modeled from both satellite and meteorological models,[40] Danesh-Yazdi and colleagues[41] reported that a warmer cold-season temperature was associated with increased respiratory disease hospitalization (rate difference = 62.13, 95% CI: 51.68, 73.02) in a large sample in the United States. There are also a commonly used gridded temperature data provided by the European Centre for Medium-Range Weather Forecasts (ECMWF) that incorporate global satellite data in their models. Although these models are spatially coarse, several studies have used the ECMWF's temperature data and reported associations between air temperature and increased risks of multiple respiratory outcomes, including respiratory disease visits[42,43] and respiratory disease mortality.[44] More recent studies have used high-resolution satellite-based modeled temperature data. For example, using the 1 km resolution temperature data modeled from MODIS satellite,[24] Yitshak-Sade and colleagues[45] reported that both short- and long-term exposure to increased ambient temperature was associated with increased respiratory disease admissions in the

Northeastern United States. Rice and colleagues[46] demonstrated that short-term average temperature exposures were associated with lower lung function. Specifically, these authors found that a 5°C increase of previous-week temperature was associated with a 20 mL lower (−34, −6) forced expiratory volume in 1 second. This effect was more pronounced in cold seasons.

AIR TEMPERATURE ENHANCED THE EFFECTS OF AIR POLLUTION ON RESPIRATORY DISEASES OUTCOMES

Emerging studies have begun investigating the synergistic health effects between these 2 exposures. In a study conducted among a Japanese population, Phosri and colleagues[47] reported strengthened associations between ambient ozone exposure and emergency ambulance dispatches when temperatures were either extremely low or extremely high. Lu and colleagues[48] linked the co-exposure to both high temperature and air pollution (eg, particulate matter with a diameter of ≤ 10 μm, PM_{10}; sulfur dioxide) with increased risk of asthma in Chinese children. Also in China, Jin and colleagues[49] reported interactions between cold weather and high fine particulate matter with a diameter of less than or equal to 2.5 μm ($PM_{2.5}$) as well as PM_{10} in relationship to increased hospitalizations of childhood asthma. This research team[50] also investigated the modifying effect of $PM_{2.5}$ on the association between temperature variability and childhood asthma hospitalizations, but no significant modifying effect was identified. Evoy and colleagues[51] conducted a panel study for the interactions between $PM_{2.5}$ and dry bulb globe temperature (DBGT) with adult lung function. Although no significant interaction was observed, the association between $PM_{2.5}$ and reduced lung functions became much stronger when DBGT was included in the models. Zhang and colleagues[52] reported that respiratory mortality was increased by 2.67% (95% CI 0.57%, 4.76%) with each 10-μg/m^3 increase in ozone (O_3) when ambient temperature exceeded 28°C. Findings from earlier studies on the interactions between ambient temperature and ambient air pollution have also been summarized in 2 review articles by Areal and colleagues[53] and Annenberg and colleagues.[54] Taken together, research to date indicates that exposure to extreme temperature amplifies the association between ambient air pollution and respiratory diseases. Moreover, this modification effect is seen as both temperature extremes, either the low temperature or the high temperature can pose increased risks of adverse respiratory outcomes.

The underlying mechanisms by which high or low temperatures may exacerbate respiratory diseases are not well understood. Airway inflammation is central to the pathophysiology of respiratory diseases including both asthma and chronic obstructive pulmonary disease[55,56] with several studies demonstrating a link between low air temperature exposure and altered inflammatory biomarkers.[57–60] Owing to the widespread interests of global warming, some studies have also investigated the mechanisms of high temperature on human health. Extremely high temperatures have been linked to increases in acute phase inflammatory biomarkers including increased platelet release and increases in red and white cell counts in circulation as a response to the heat exposure.[61] How changes in these acute phase response indicators are related to respiratory diseases are not clear. Other research suggest that high air temperature may affect the systemic thermoregulation and thereby lead to airway inflammation.[62–64] Besides the direct and acute impact of air temperature on the human body, warming temperatures related to climate change can increase the formation of O_3 and ambient aeroallergens[65] (eg, pollens), further impact respiratory heath.

SUMMARY

Existing and evolving methods increasingly provide highly spatially and temporally resolved exposure data relevant to climate research in respiratory health. This review focuses on an exemplary approach leveraging advances in satellite remote sensing coupled with advanced geospatial modeling approaches to characterize temperature exposures. These new modeling methods and algorithms advance the state of the art in epidemiological studies looking at the respiratory health effects of climate change and increase the number of subjects for which exposure estimates are available globally.

These methods have enabled research that contributes to a growing evidence base linking temperature extremes (hot and cold) with adverse respiratory outcomes. More mechanistic studies are needed to understand the biological underpinnings of these associations. Additionally, studies examining the complex interactions among temperature, air pollution, and aeroallergen exposures are worthy of more exploration to elucidate the fuller scope of climate change effects on respiratory health. Unless strategies are put in place to curb global climate change, we will continue to see upward trends in both acute and chronic respiratory health impacts.

CLINICS CARE POINTS

- The rise in global temperature has led to an increase in heat waves and extreme weather events, which pose serious risks to respiratory health and can lead to worsened symptoms for patients with respiratory diseases.

- Recent advances in open-source earth observations data have allowed for improved exposure assessment through temperature modeling, which can provide clinics with more accurate data to inform clinical decisions.

- Spatio-temporally resolved air temperature data at the residence scale can reduce exposure bias and enhance our understanding of the immediate health consequences associated with ambient temperature, which can inform treatment plans and improve patient outcomes.

- Clinics can play a crucial role in mitigating the effects of climate change on respiratory health by implementing appropriate measures, such as educating patients on how to protect themselves during extreme weather events and high temperature periods.

ACKNOWLEDGMENTS

During preparation of this article, I. Kloog and X. Zhang were supported by National Institutes of Health (NIH) Grants UG3/H3OD023337, P30ES023515, and UL1TR004419.

DISCLOSURE/CONFLICTS OF INTEREST

There are no conflicts of interest.

REFERENCES

1. McMichael AJ, Wilkinson P, Kovats RS, et al. International study of temperature, heat and urban mortality: the 'ISOTHURM' project. Int J Epidemiol 2008;37(5): 1121–31.
2. IPCC, 2023: *Climate Change 2023: Synthesis Report*. A Report of the Intergovernmental Panel on Climate Change. Contribution of Working Groups I, II and III to the

Sixth Assessment Report of the Intergovernmental Panel on Climate Change, Core Writing Team, Lee H and Romero J, (eds.). IPCC, Geneva, Switzerland, (in press).

3. Satterthwaite D. The implications of population growth and urbanization for climate change. Environ Urbanization 2009;21(2):545–67.

4. Hughes L. Biological consequences of global warming: is the signal already apparent? Trends Ecol Evol 2000;15(2):56–61.

5. Basu R, Samet JM. Relation between elevated ambient temperature and mortality: a review of the epidemiologic evidence. Epidemiol Rev 2002;24(2):190–202.

6. Robine J-M, Cheung SLK, Le Roy S, et al. Death toll exceeded 70,000 in Europe during the summer of 2003. Comptes Rendus Biol 2008;331(2):171–8.

7. Tan J, Zheng Y, Tang X, et al. The urban heat island and its impact on heat waves and human health in Shanghai. Int J Biometeorol 2010;54(1):75–84.

8. Guo Y, Gasparrini A, Armstrong B, et al. Global variation in the effects of ambient temperature on mortality: a systematic evaluation. Epidemiology 2014;25(6): 781–9.

9. Gasparrini A, Guo Y, Hashizume M, et al. Mortality risk attributable to high and low ambient temperature: a multicountry observational study. Lancet 2015; 386(9991):369–75.

10. Song X, Wang S, Hu Y, et al. Impact of ambient temperature on morbidity and mortality: an overview of reviews. Sci Total Environ 2017;586:241–54.

11. Cheng J, Xu Z, Zhu R, et al. Impact of diurnal temperature range on human health: a systematic review. Int J Biometeorol 2014;58(9):2011–24.

12. Bunker A, Wildenhain J, Vandenbergh A, et al. Effects of air temperature on climate-sensitive mortality and morbidity outcomes in the elderly; a systematic review and meta-analysis of epidemiological evidence. EBioMedicine 2016;6: 258–68.

13. Vanos JK. Children's health and vulnerability in outdoor microclimates: a comprehensive review. Environ Int 2015;76:1–15.

14. Stewart S, Keates AK, Redfern A, et al. Seasonal variations in cardiovascular disease. Nat Rev Cardiol 2017;14(11):654–64.

15. Wu X, Lu Y, Zhou S, et al. Impact of climate change on human infectious diseases: Empirical evidence and human adaptation. Environ Int 2016;86:14–23.

16. Stafoggia M, Schwartz J, Forastiere F, et al. Does temperature modify the association between air pollution and mortality? A multicity case-crossover analysis in Italy. Am J Epidemiol 2008;167(12):1476–85.

17. Zeger SL, Thomas D, Dominici F, et al. Exposure measurement error in time-series studies of air pollution: concepts and consequences. Environ Health Perspect 2000;108(5):419–26.

18. Sergio MV-S, Saz-SÃƒÂ¡nchez MA, JosÃƒÂ© MC. Comparative analysis of interpolation methods in the middle Ebro Valley (Spain): application to annual precipitation and temperature. Clim Res 2003;24(2):161–80.

19. Tsin PK, Knudby A, Krayenhoff ES, et al. Land use regression modeling of microscale urban air temperatures in greater Vancouver, Canada. Urban Clim 2020;32: 100636.

20. Burger M, Gubler M, Heinimann A, et al. Modelling the spatial pattern of heatwaves in the city of Bern using a land use regression approach. Urban Clim 2021;38:100885.

21. Janatian N, Sadeghi M, Sanaeinejad SH, et al. A statistical framework for estimating air temperature using MODIS land surface temperature data. Int J Climatol 2017;37(3):1181–94.

22. Li Z-L, Wu H, Wang N, et al. Land surface emissivity retrieval from satellite data. Int J Rem Sens 2013;34(9–10):3084–127.
23. Kloog I, Chudnovsky A, Koutrakis P, et al. Temporal and spatial assessments of minimum air temperature using satellite surface temperature measurements in Massachusetts, USA. Sci Total Environ 2012;432:85–92.
24. Kloog I, Nordio F, Coull BA, et al. Predicting spatiotemporal mean air temperature using MODIS satellite surface temperature measurements across the Northeastern USA. Remote Sens Environ 2014;150:132–9.
25. Shi L, Liu P, Kloog I, et al. Estimating daily air temperature across the Southeastern United States using high-resolution satellite data: a statistical modeling study. Environ Res 2016;146:51–8.
26. Kloog I, Nordio F, Lepeule J, et al. Modelling spatio-temporally resolved air temperature across the complex geo-climate area of France using satellite-derived land surface temperature data. Int J Climatol 2017;37(1):296–304.
27. Wan Z. New refinements and validation of the collection-6 MODIS land-surface temperature/emissivity product. Remote Sens Environ 2014;140:36–45.
28. Xue J, Anderson MC, Gao F, et al. Sharpening ECOSTRESS and VIIRS land surface temperature using harmonized Landsat-Sentinel surface reflectances. Remote Sens Environ 2020;251:112055.
29. Voogt JA, Oke TR. Complete urban surface temperatures. J Appl Meteorol 1997;36(9):1117–32.
30. Vancutsem C, Ceccato P, Dinku T, et al. Evaluation of MODIS land surface temperature data to estimate air temperature in different ecosystems over Africa. Remote Sens Environ 2010;114(2):449–65.
31. Jin M, Dickinson RE. Land surface skin temperature climatology: benefitting from the strengths of satellite observations. Environ Res Lett 2010;5(4):044004.
32. Zhou B, Erell E, Hough I, et al. Estimation of hourly near surface air temperature across Israel using an ensemble model. Rem Sens 2020;12(11):1741.
33. Oyler JW, Ballantyne A, Jencso K, et al. Creating a topoclimatic daily air temperature dataset for the conterminous United States using homogenized station data and remotely sensed land skin temperature. Int J Climatol 2015;35(9):2258–79
34. Hough I, Just AC, Zhou B, et al. A multi-resolution air temperature model for France from MODIS and Landsat thermal data. Environ Res 2020;183:109244.
35. Jin Z, Ma Y, Chu L, et al. Predicting spatiotemporally-resolved mean air temperature over Sweden from satellite data using an ensemble model. Environ Res 2022;204:111960.
36. Flückiger B, Kloog I, Ragettli MS, et al. Modelling daily air temperature at a fine spatial resolution dealing with challenging meteorological phenomena and topography in Switzerland. Int J Climatol 2022;42(12):6413–28.
37. Du R, Jiao W, Ma J, et al. Association between ambient temperature and chronic rhinosinusitis. Int Forum Allergy Rhinol 2023;1–9. https://doi.org/10.1002/alr.23152.
38. Chen Y, Kong D, Fu J, et al. Associations between ambient temperature and adult asthma hospitalizations in Beijing, China: a time-stratified case-crossover study. Respir Res 2022;23(1):38.
39. Green RS, Basu R, Malig B, et al. The effect of temperature on hospital admissions in nine California counties. Int J Publ Health 2010;55(2):113–21.
40. Abatzoglou JT. Development of gridded surface meteorological data for ecological applications and modelling. Int J Climatol 2013;33(1):121–31.
41. Danesh Yazdi M, Wei Y, Di Q, et al. The effect of long-term exposure to air pollution and seasonal temperature on hospital admissions with cardiovascular and

respiratory disease in the United States: a difference-in-differences analysis. Sci Total Environ 2022;843:156855.

42. Wanka ER, Bayerstadler A, Heumann C, et al. Weather and air pollutants have an impact on patients with respiratory diseases and breathing difficulties in Munich, Germany. Int J Biometeorol 2014;58(2):249–62.

43. Ferrari U, Exner T, Wanka ER, et al. Influence of air pressure, humidity, solar radiation, temperature, and wind speed on ambulatory visits due to chronic obstructive pulmonary disease in Bavaria, Germany. Int J Biometeorol 2012;56(1):137–43.

44. Jacobson LdSV, Oliveira BF Ad, Schneider R, et al. Mortality risk from respiratory diseases due to non-optimal temperature among brazilian elderlies. Int J Environ Res Publ Health 2021;18(11):5550.

45. Yitshak-Sade M, Bobb JF, Schwartz JD, et al. The association between short and long-term exposure to PM2.5 and temperature and hospital admissions in New England and the synergistic effect of the short-term exposures. Sci Total Environ 2018;639:868–75.

46. Rice MB, Li W, Wilker EH, et al. Association of outdoor temperature with lung function in a temperate climate. Eur Respir J 2019;53(1):1800612.

47. Phosri A, Ueda K, Seposo X, et al. Effect modification by temperature on the association between O3 and emergency ambulance dispatches in Japan: a multi-city study. Sci Total Environ 2023;861:160725.

48. Lu C, Zhang Y, Li B, et al. Interaction effect of prenatal and postnatal exposure to ambient air pollution and temperature on childhood asthma. Environ Int 2022;167:107456.

49. Jin X, Xu Z, Liang Y, et al. The modification of air particulate matter on the relationship between temperature and childhood asthma hospitalization: an exploration based on different interaction strategies. Environ Res 2022;214:113848.

50. Yan S, Wang X, Yao Z, et al. Seasonal characteristics of temperature variability impacts on childhood asthma hospitalization in Hefei, China: does PM2.5 modify the association? Environ Res 2022;207:112078.

51. Evoy R, Kincl L, Rohlman D, et al. Impact of acute temperature and air pollution exposures on adult lung function: a panel study of asthmatics. PLoS One 2022;17(6):e0270412.

52. Zhang Y, Tian Q, Feng X, et al. Modification effects of ambient temperature on ozone-mortality relationships in Chengdu, China. Environ Sci Pollut Control Ser 2022;29(48):73011–9.

53. Areal AT, Zhao Q, Wigmann C, et al. The effect of air pollution when modified by temperature on respiratory health outcomes: a systematic review and meta-analysis. Sci Total Environ 2022;811:152336.

54. Anenberg SC, Haines S, Wang E, et al. Synergistic health effects of air pollution, temperature, and pollen exposure: a systematic review of epidemiological evidence. Environ Health 2020;19(1):130.

55. Saetta M. Airway inflammation in chronic obstructive pulmonary disease. Am J Respir Crit Care Med 1999;160(supplement_1):S17–20.

56. Wardlaw AJ, Brightling CE, Green R, et al. New insights into the relationship between airway inflammation and asthma. Clin Sci 2002;103(2):201–11.

57. Peters A, Panagiotakos D, Picciotto S, et al. Air temperature and inflammatory responses in myocardial infarction survivors. Epidemiology 2008;19(3):391–400.

58. Halonen JI, Zanobetti A, Sparrow D, et al. Associations between outdoor temperature and markers of inflammation: a cohort study. Environ Health 2010;9(1):42.

59. Larsson K, Tornling G, Gavhed D, et al. Inhalation of cold air increases the number of inflammatory cells in the lungs in healthy subjects. Eur Respir J 1998;12(4): 825–30.
60. Schäuble CL, Hampel R, Breitner S, et al. Short-term effects of air temperature on blood markers of coagulation and inflammation in potentially susceptible individuals. Occup Environ Med 2012;69(9):670–8.
61. Keatinge WR, Coleshaw SRK, Easton JC, et al. Increased platelet and red cell counts, blood viscosity, and plasma cholesterol levels during heat stress, and mortality from coronary and cerebral thrombosis. Am J Med 1986;81(5):795–800.
62. Deng L, Ma P, Wu Y, et al. High and low temperatures aggravate airway inflammation of asthma: evidence in a mouse model. Environ Pollut 2020;256:113433.
63. Sprung CL, Portocarrero CJ, Fernaine AV, et al. The metabolic and respiratory alterations of heat stroke. Arch Intern Med 1980;140(5):665–9.
64. Bouchama A, De Vol EB. Acid-base alterations in heatstroke. Intensive Care Med 2001;27(4):680–5.
65. Beggs PJ. Impacts of climate change on aeroallergens: past and future. Clin Exp Allergy 2004;34(10):1507–13.

Clinical Medicine and Climate Change

Pablo E. Morejón-Jaramillo, MD, Nicholas J. Nassikas, MD,
Mary B. Rice, MD, MPH*

KEYWORDS

- Climate change • Air pollution • Greenhouse gas emissions • Greenhouse effect
- CO_2 emissions • Physician-patient relationship • Improving health care

KEY POINTS

- Clinical medicine can contribute to climate change.
- Extreme weather impairs health care delivery.
- Clinicians can counsel patients on climate-related health effects.

INTRODUCTION

Climate change is one of the greatest threats to public health today. As reviewed elsewhere in this series, increasing global temperatures have influenced the spread of infectious diseases, contributed to worsening air pollution, magnified global eco-anxiety, prolonged and intensified the pollen season, and led to heat waves that can independently and jointly affect patients with asthma. The changes in climate we are experiencing are the result of human-related activities, primarily emissions of greenhouse gases from burning fossil fuels. As a result of continued dependence on fossil fuels for energy, these events are anticipated to worsen in the future if not intervened on. Thus, clinicians need to be aware of climate-related impacts on respiratory health in order to better counsel patients on health effects and help mitigate risks.

Not only do we need to learn to respond as health care providers, we also need to understand how the health care industry can also be a potential contributor to global greenhouse gas emissions from activities such as the transportation of staff, patients, and medical supplies as well as the production of energy to power hospitals and clinics. Fossil fuel–derived air pollution impairs the health of nearby communities served by health care systems but also has more widespread health implications through influences on climate change. Moreover, consequences of climate change

Division of Pulmonary and Critical Care Medicine, Department of Medicine, Beth Israel Deaconess Medical Center, 330 Brookline Avenue, Boston, MA 02215-5491, USA
* Corresponding author.
E-mail address: mrice1@bidmc.harvard.edu

Immunol Allergy Clin N Am 44 (2024) 109–117
https://doi.org/10.1016/j.iac.2023.07.006
0889-8561/24/© 2023 Elsevier Inc. All rights reserved.

including extreme weather events, such as floods, hurricanes, and wildfires, can impede people's ability to obtain essential medical care through disruptions in transportation and other effects.

This article highlights 4 elements to consider regarding the intersection of clinical medicine and climate change with particular focus on respiratory health care implications. The authors describe (1) how clinical medicine potentially contributes to climate change, (2) how extreme weather impairs health care delivery, and (3) how clinicians can guide patients on the health effects of climate change and ways to mitigate risks and (4) highlight emerging efforts in climate and health education to ensure we have the workforce needed to respond to urgent ongoing and emerging health challenges to climate change.

Raising Awareness of Contribution of Clinical Medicine to Climate Change

It is increasingly recognized that health care systems both in the United States (US) and abroad can be significant contributors to greenhouse gas emissions, responsible for 5% to 8% of the global greenhouse gas emissions[1-4]; this has led to a growing interest in reducing the carbon footprint of health care systems and institutions. Emissions are generated throughout the system, either directly from health care operations (7%), indirectly from electricity usage (11%), or indirectly from supply-chain activities such as transportation (eg, for patients, for staff, for goods and services) and manufacturing (eg, medical products, chemicals, gases) (82%).[4] The supply chain category accounts for most of the greenhouse gas emissions and is also known as Scope 3—the indirect costs on which the health care system depends but does not directly own or control. Included in Scope 3 are pharmaceuticals and chemicals (18% of the total health care greenhouse gas emissions); medical supplies and devices (7%); food, water, and waste (12%) transport, for instance by health care workers who comprise one of the largest commuting workforces in the US (4%).[4-6]

A potentially less recognized source of greenhouse gas emissions within health care results from 2 drug classes, anesthetics and meter-dose inhalers for lung disease. Anesthetics used for sedation during medical procedures are potent greenhouse gases.[7,8] The principal anesthetics causing this harm are isoflurane, sevoflurane, and desflurane, the latter having particular global warming potential.[7-10] In 2014, these anesthetics produced 3 million tons of carbon dioxide, of which 80% were due to desflurane. Halothane was also included in this category in the 1960s, but it has since been phased out in developing countries due to adverse effects on the liver.[8] There are no mechanisms in existence right now to capture anesthetic gases when they are used[8]; this is particularly concerning because the atmospheric lifetime of sevoflurane, isoflurane, desflurane, and N_2O can be up to 5, 6, 21, and 114 years, respectively.[9,11]

Even more relevant to the current discussion, an increasingly recognized source of greenhouse gas emissions is the use of metered dose inhalers (MDIs) for respiratory conditions. MDIs use hydrofluorocarbons, a potent greenhouse gas, as a propellant to deliver the medication. On the other hand, dry powder inhalers (DPIs) do not use a propellant and may offer providers and patients an alternative choice. Research is beginning to directly examine how transitioning from an MDI to a DPI for maintenance asthma therapy can reduce the heat-trapping emissions of inhaler use, with a recent study documenting benefits relative to climate emissions without compromising asthma control.[12] Specifically, patients switching from a pressurized MDI to DPI-based maintenance therapy more than halved their inhaler carbon footprint without loss of asthma control. These findings in part informed guidance to consider the lower carbon footprint of DPIs alongside other factors when choosing inhalation devices for asthma management. Although DPIs may be an acceptable alternative in terms of efficacy, some children, elderly, and patients with chronic lung disease may have a harder time using DPIs.[12,13]

Extreme Weather Effects on Health Care Delivery

Climate change is increasing the frequency and intensity of extreme weather events across the world with implications for clinical medicine, particularly access to care. Extreme weather events are a major and unpredictable hazard to the delivery of health care. Each step along the way, from the manufacturing and shipment of drugs and medical supplies, to the provision of care to patients in clinics and hospitals is at risk of interruption.

Extreme weather events impede access to hospitals and health care systems and hinder the delivery of care to patients in a variety of ways. For example, extreme weather events, which are becoming more common due to climate change, can cause substantial damage to medical infrastructure and facilities.[14] A striking historical example of such disruption is Hurricane Katrina, which made landfall over New Orleans in August 2005, severely affecting the regional health care system. Among the affected medical facilities were Tulane Medical Center, Charity, and University Hospitals, which were forced to cease operations.[15,16] The hurricane disproportionately affected low-income communities who relied on these hospitals for medical care.[15,16]

The disproportionate impact on already vulnerable populations has been seen globally. Flooding events across the world, including the Far East, have forced hospitals to shut down and patients to be relocated to alternative health facilities, adding particular stress to systems already suffering from a lack of hospital beds and medical personnel.[17,18] When patients are evacuated from health care facilities or relocated due to climate-related extreme weather events, the environmental health threats to underlying chronic conditions such as asthma discussed elsewhere in this series are compounded by consequent risk of interruptions in their medications.[19] Extreme weather events such as flooding have obstructed access to rural health centers[20] and may have longer lasting effects in light of cooccurring health challenges facing those in more remote regions of the world. Rural and aboriginal communities are further affected when primary health centers are converted to evacuation or distribution centers and thus become nonoperational in delivering health care.[14]

In addition, extreme weather conditions can also disrupt access to medications and pharmacies.[21] In the aftermath of Hurricane Katrina, some diabetic patients lost access to insulin, and schizophrenic and bipolar patients were unable to obtain prescription drugs for up to 6 months after the hurricane.[16]

Extreme weather events can also interfere with the supply chain for medications. In September 2017, Hurricane Maria made landfall over Puerto Rico, causing shortages in intravenous saline solution production that affected the US health care system, as Puerto Rico was a major producer of saline solution.[22] The hurricane also caused shortages in immunosuppressive medications that were manufactured in Puerto Rico.[15,23–25] The earthquake that affected the Tohoku region in Japan in 2011 also destroyed 10 hospitals and damaged more than 500 hospitals along with critical medical facilities, contributing to further shortages in essential medications.[26,27]

Lessons learned from the health care challenges experienced following such climate-related events emphasize the need to build more resilient health care delivery systems that will optimally respond to future extreme weather events.

Clinical Guidance for Patients

Health care providers can play an important role in helping patients avoid or minimize the effects of climate change on their health. Interventions include[1] describing the link between common environmental triggers, climate change, and health (eg, mold, pollen, smoke),[2] counseling patients on medications that might increase their risk to heat, and[3] suggesting ways of mitigating exposure to smoke and aeroallergens (eg, N95 face masks or HEPA filters). Educating patients on environmental risks to their health, reviewing their medications, and offering interventions such as face masks and respirators are ways in which clinicians can help guide patients as they face increasingly frequent climate-related health hazards.

An important first step is to describe the link between climate change and common environmental triggers to help patients anticipate environmental changes that may affect their health. Patients view physicians as a trustworthy source of information for various complicated subjects. Therefore, providing them with accurate information about climate change and its impact on their symptoms can improve communication regarding this matter.[28] One such example, which affects a large proportion of the population with allergic rhinitis or allergic asthma, is how climate change is prolonging pollen seasons and increasing pollen concentrations within the pollen season.[15,29–31] As pollen is a common trigger of allergic rhinitis and asthma symptoms, patients may decide to change their behavior to adapt to these changes with counseling from their providers.

Wildfires are another example for which clinicians can provide guidance. Wildfires are increasing in intensity and frequency across the globe as a result of climate change.[32] There are thousands of chemicals in wildfire smoke.[33] The smoke from wildfires can exacerbate chronic lung diseases, especially asthma, but also chronic obstructive pulmonary disease (COPD)[34] and cardiovascular disease.[35] Plumes of wildfire smoke particles, consisting of thousands of chemicals, can travel to distant places, affecting the respiratory health of communities who live far from the fire, and often times the smoke from multiple fires burning simultaneously can severely impair air quality for an entire region.[36] As one recent example, in June 2023 (at the time of this writing), Canadian fires caused several days of hazardous air quality conditions in major cities across the East Coast of US.[37]

Extreme heat is a third major climate-related exposure that warrants clinical guidance. Populations susceptible to heat-related health effects include children,[38,39] the elderly, and those with underlying chronic lung or heart disease.[40] Racially/ethnically minoritized and low-income communities may be differentially exposed to extreme heat due to the urban heat island effect and reduced access to air conditioning. In addition, certain medications can increase susceptibility to heat-related health effects, by causing dehydration, increasing intrinsic heat production, or impairing the body's ability to thermoregulate. These medications include anticholinergics/antimuscarinics, diuretics, and stimulants.[41,42] Patients using these medications may have more difficulty coping with heat waves and may benefit from counseling on heat adaptation.

In the face of multiple climate change–related health threats, there are interventions that may help reduce exposure (**Table 1**). HEPA air purifiers reduce levels of indoor air pollutants and aeroallergens. In nonwildfire settings, the use of air purifiers has been found to reduce symptoms and improve lung function in patients with asthma and allergies and improve symptoms in COPD.[43–48] Unfortunately, HEPA filters may not be accessible for everyone due to high costs for the machine or reliable and affordable power supplies. N95 face masks can filter out air pollutants and aeroallergens and may be suitable for short-term use (eg, commuting or evacuating during wildfire smoke events) although not practical to wear at all times. Air conditioning is likely the most effective intervention for extreme heat but also presents issues of cost and access.[49] Use of fans is a lower cost alternative but with lower

Table 1
Climate change–related health threats

Climate-Related Exposures	Interventions to Reduce Exposure and Health Effects
Pollen	• Taking antiallergy medications (eg, antihistamines, nasal decongestants)[52] • Use of HEPA air purifiers • Avoiding outdoor activities when pollen levels are high • Nocturnal laminar airflow device for patients with asthma[52]
Wildfire smoke	• Use of HEPA air purifiers[34,53] • Minimizing outdoor activity during smoke events • Closing windows and doors • Wearing N95 masks (if feasible) for unavoidable high-exposure intervals[34]
Extreme heat and heat waves	• Staying hydrated • Avoiding outdoor activities during high temperatures[54] • Wearing loose and light color clothes • Use of fans[50] or air conditioners[55] • Traveling to a community cooling center[56] • Adhering to warning systems and developing prevention plans[57]
Combustion-related pollution	• Using HEPA air purifiers[58] • Minimizing outdoor activity during air quality alerts
Floods and mold production	• Use of ventilation and air condition systems to reduce indoor humidity and minimize mold growth[51] • Use of dehumidifiers to minimize mold growth[51] • Housing accommodations (if feasible) to avoid living on ground or basement level[59,60]

cooling potential.[50] Installation of dehumidifiers and creating buildings that are protected against floods may help decrease mold formation, which can trigger asthma symptoms.[51] **Table 1** describes potential interventions that the clinician can discuss with patients to help mitigate the health effects of climate change. In each case, there is a need for more formal clinical guidelines and measures to ensure equitable access.[52–60]

Climate and Health Education

We must also be focused on workforce development, ensuring that we have the capacity to respond to the health care challenges stemming from climate change. Developing curricula that disseminate the existing evidence base for climate change–driven impacts on human health is crucial for preparing future practitioners to identify and address these impacts.

SUMMARY

The impact of climate change on clinical care is evident through its interference with access to health care and the adverse health effects of extreme heat, floods, wildfire smoke, pollen, consequent eco-anxiety, and other climate-related exposures. Health care providers can address the health crisis caused by climate change by advocating for more sustainable health care delivery systems as well as directly helping patients anticipate potential health impacts and reduce their exposure to these hazards. We also need to expand efforts to train the workforce needed to provide quality and effective health care in the face of unique challenges in this context.

CLINICS CARE POINTS

- Patients with with advanced age, environmental allergies and chronic respiratory disease are at high risk of advsere health effects of climate-related airborne hazards
- Clinicians can counsel patients on interventions to mitigate the health effects of pollen, wildfire smoke, extreme heat, combustion pollution and mold (Table 1)

DISCLOSURE

Dr M.B. Rice reports receiving grants from the NIH, United States and payments from the Conservation Law Foundation, unrelated to the submitted work.

REFERENCES

1. Thiel C, Richie C. Carbon Emissions from Overuse of U.S. Health Care: Medical and Ethical Problems. Hastings Cent Rep 2022;52(4):10–6.
2. Tennison I, Roschnik S, Ashby B, et al. Health care's response to climate change: a carbon footprint assessment of the NHS in England. Lancet Planet Health 2021; 5(2):e84–92.
3. Karliner J, Slotterback S, Boyd R, et al. Health care's climate footprint: the health sector contribution and opportunities for action. Eur J Public Health 2020; 30(Supplement_5). ckaa165.843.
4. Eckelman MJ, Huang K, Lagasse R, et al. Health Care Pollution And Public Health Damage In The United States: An Update: Study examines health care pollution and public health damage in the United States. Health Aff 2020;39(12):2071–9.
5. Priceonomics. Which Professions Have the Longest Commutes? Internet. Priceonomics. 2016. Available at: https://priceonomics.com/which-professions-have-the-longest-commutes/. Accessed June 9, 2023.
6. Sampath B, Jensen M, Lenoci-Edwards J, et al. Reducing Healthcare Carbon Emissions: A Primer on Measures and Actions for Healthcare Organizations to Mitigate Climate Change. (Prepared by Institute for Healthcare Improvement under Contract No. 75Q80122P00007.) AHRQ Publication No. 22-M011. Rockville, MD: Agency for Healthcare Research and Quality; 2022.
7. Charlesworth M, Swinton F. Anaesthetic gases, climate change, and sustainable practice. Lancet Planet Health 2017;1(6):e216–7.
8. Vollmer MK, Rhee TS, Rigby M, et al. Modern inhalation anesthetics: Potent greenhouse gases in the global atmosphere. Geophys Res Lett 2015;42(5): 1606–11.
9. Roizen MF. Global Warming Potential of Inhaled Anesthetics: Application to Clinical Use. Yearb Anesthesiol Pain Manag 2011;2011:13–4.
10. Wyssusek K, Chan KL, Eames G, et al. Greenhouse gas reduction in anaesthesia practice: a departmental environmental strategy. BMJ Open Qual 2022;11(3): e001867.
11. Varughese S, Ahmed R. Environmental and Occupational Considerations of Anesthesia: A Narrative Review and Update. Anesth Analg 2021;133(4):826–35.
12. Woodcock A, Janson C, Rees J, et al. Effects of switching from a metered dose inhaler to a dry powder inhaler on climate emissions and asthma control: post-hoc analysis. Thorax 2022;77(12):1187–92.
13. Ye Y, Ma Y, Zhu J. The future of dry powder inhaled therapy: Promising or discouraging for systemic disorders? Int J Pharm 2022;614:121457.

14. Lal A, Patel M, Hunter A, et al. Towards resilient health systems for increasing climate extremes: insights from the 2019–20 Australian bushfire season. Int J Wildland Fire 2021;30(1):1.

15. Shankar HM, Rice MB. Update on Climate Change. Clin Chest Med 2020;41(4): 753–61.

16. Rudowitz R, Rowland D, Shartzer A. Health Care In New Orleans Before And After Hurricane Katrina: The storm of 2005 exposed problems that had existed for years and made solutions more complex and difficult to obtain. Health Aff 2006;25(Suppl1):W393–406.

17. France-Presse A. Malaysia's worst flooding in years leaves 30,000 people displaced. The Guardian Internet. 2021 Dec 19; Available at: https://www.theguardian.com/world/2021/dec/19/malaysias-worst-flooding-in-years-leaves-30000-people-displaced. Accessed May 8, 2023.

18. Yusoff NA, Shafii H, Omar R. The impact of floods in hospital and mitigation measures: A literature review. IOP Conf Ser Mater Sci Eng 2017;271:012026.

19. Tomio J, Sato H, Mizumura H. Interruption of Medication among Outpatients with Chronic Conditions after a Flood. Prehospital Disaster Med 2010;25(1):42–50.

20. Sarkar S. Pakistan floods pose serious health challenges. BMJ 2022;o2141.

21. Ochi S, Hodgson S, Landeg O, et al. Disaster-Driven Evacuation and Medication Loss: a Systematic Literature Review. PLoS Curr 2014;6. ecurrents.dis.fa417630 b566a0c7dfdbf945910edd96.

22. Sacks CA, Kesselheim AS, Fralick M. The Shortage of Normal Saline in the Wake of Hurricane Maria. JAMA Intern Med 2018;178(7):885–6.

23. Pullen LC. Puerto Rico after Hurricane Maria. Am J Transplant 2018;18(2):283–4.

24. Wong JC. Hospitals face critical shortage of IV bags due to Puerto Rico hurricane. The Guardian Internet. 2018 . Available at: https://www.theguardian.com/us-news/2018/jan/10/hurricane-maria-puerto-rico-iv-bag-shortage-hospitals. Accessed May 8, 2023.

25. Guerra Velázquez GR. Hurricane María and Public Health in Puerto Rico: Lessons Learned to Increase Resiliency and Prepare for Future Disasters. Ann Glob Health 2022;88(1):82.

26. Learning-from-Megadisasters-lessons-from-the-great-east-Japan-earthquake.pdf \ Internet. Available at: https://documents1.worldbank.org/curated/en/478711468 038957554/pdf/Learning-from-Megadisasters-lessons-from-the-great-east-Japan-earthquake.pdf. Accessed May 10, 2023.

27. Yokobori Y, Sakai T, Takeda T, Oi T. Post Earthquake Health Information Management in Japan—the Challenges. Perspect Health Inf Manag Internet. 2015 May;(International issue). Available at: http://library.ahima.org/doc?oid=301178. Accessed May 10, 2023.

28. Senay E, Sarfaty M, Rice MB. Strategies for Clinical Discussions About Climate Change. Ann Intern Med 2021;174(3):417–8.

29. D'Amato G, Vitale C, Rosario N, et al. Climate change, allergy and asthma, and the role of tropical forests. World Allergy Organ J 2017;10(1):11.

30. D'Amato G, Cecchi L, D'Amato M, et al. Climate change and respiratory diseases. Eur Respir Rev 2014;23(132):161–9.

31. Deng SZ, Jalaludin BB, Antó JM, et al. Climate change, air pollution, and allergic respiratory diseases: a call to action for health professionals. Chin Med J (Engl) 2020;133(13):1552–60.

32. Wu Y, Li S, Xu R, et al. Wildfire-related PM2.5 and health economic loss of mortality in Brazil. Environ Int 2023;174:107906.

33. Balmes JR. The Changing Nature of Wildfires: Impacts on the Health of the Public. Clin Chest Med 2020;41(4):771–6.
34. Rice MB, Henderson SB, Lambert AA, et al. Respiratory Impacts of Wildland Fire Smoke: Future Challenges and Policy Opportunities. An Official American Thoracic Society Workshop Report. Ann Am Thorac Soc 2021;18(6):921–30.
35. Cascio WE. Wildland Fire Smoke and Human Health. Sci Total Environ 2018;624: 586–95.
36. Canon G, Kamal R. What the numbers tells us about a catastrophic year of wildfires. The Guardian Internet. 2021 Dec 25; Available at: https://www.theguardian.com/us-news/2021/dec/25/what-the-numbers-tells-us-about-a-catastrophic-year-of-wildfires. Accessed Jun 8, 2023.
37. Dong M, Malsky B, Bloch M, Gómez MG, Jones J, Murphy JM, et al. Maps: Tracking Air Quality and Smoke From Canada Wildfires. The New York Times Internet. 2023 Jun 7; Available at: https://www.nytimes.com/interactive/2023/us/smoke-maps-canada-fires.html. Accessed Jun 8, 2023.
38. Smith CJ. Pediatric Thermoregulation: Considerations in the Face of Global Climate Change. Nutrients 2019;11(9):2010.
39. Uibel D, Sharma R, Piontkowski D, et al. Association of Ambient Extreme Heat with Pediatric Morbidity: A Scoping Review. Int J Biometeorol 2022;66(8):1683–98.
40. Kenny GP, Yardley J, Brown C, et al. Heat stress in older individuals and patients with common chronic diseases. CMAJ Can Med Assoc J 2010;182(10):1053–60.
41. Levine M, LoVecchio F, Ruha AM, et al. Influence of Drug Use on Morbidity and Mortality in Heatstroke. J Med Toxicol 2012;8(3):252–7.
42. McAllen KJ, Schwartz DR. Adverse drug reactions resulting in hyperthermia in the intensive care unit. Crit Care Med 2010;38:S244.
43. Hansel NN, Putcha N, Woo H, et al. Randomized Clinical Trial of Air Cleaners to Improve Indoor Air Quality and Chronic Obstructive Pulmonary Disease Health: Results of the CLEAN AIR Study. Am J Respir Crit Care Med 2022;205(4):421–30.
44. Park HK, Cheng KC, Tetteh AO, et al. Effectiveness of air purifier on health outcomes and indoor particles in homes of children with allergic diseases in Fresno, California: A pilot study. J Asthma 2017;54(4):341–6.
45. Park HJ, Lee HY, Suh CH, et al. The Effect of Particulate Matter Reduction by Indoor Air Filter Use on Respiratory Symptoms and Lung Function: A Systematic Review and Meta-analysis. Allergy Asthma Immunol Res 2021;13(5):719–32.
46. Vesper SJ, Wymer L, Coull BA, et al. HEPA filtration intervention in classrooms may improve some students' asthma. J Asthma 2023;60(3):479–86.
47. McDonald E, Cook D, Newman T, et al. Effect of Air Filtration Systems on Asthma. Chest 2002;122(5):1535–42.
48. van Boven FE, de Jong NW, Braunstahl GJ, et al. Effectiveness of the Air Purification Strategies for the Treatment of Allergic Asthma: A Meta-Analysis. Int Arch Allergy Immunol 2020;181(5):395–402.
49. Colelli FP, Wing IS, Cian ED. Air-conditioning adoption and electricity demand highlight climate change mitigation–adaptation tradeoffs. Sci Rep 2023;13:4413.
50. Jay O, Cramer MN, Ravanelli NM, et al. Should electric fans be used during a heat wave? Appl Ergon 2015;46:137–43.
51. Seppänen O, Kurnitski J. Moisture control and ventilation. In: WHO Guidelines for Indoor Air Quality: Dampness and Mould Internet. World Health Organization; 2009 cited 2023 May 26. Available from: https://www.ncbi.nlm.nih.gov/books/NBK143947/.

52. Kapoor M, Storrar W, Balls L, et al. Nocturnal temperature-controlled laminar airflow device for adults with severe allergic asthma: the LASER RCT. Health Technol Assess Winch Engl 2019;23(29):1–140.
53. Barn PK, Elliott CT, Allen RW, et al. Portable air cleaners should be at the forefront of the public health response to landscape fire smoke. Environ Health 2016; 15:116.
54. Gauer R, Meyers BK. Heat-Related Illnesses. Am Fam Physician 2019;99(8): 482–9.
55. Milando CW, Black-Ingersoll F, Heidari L, et al. Mixed methods assessment of personal heat exposure, sleep, physical activity, and heat adaptation strategies among urban residents in the Boston area, MA. BMC Publ Health 2022;22:2314.
56. Kim K, Jung J, Schollaert C, et al. A Comparative Assessment of Cooling Center Preparedness across Twenty-Five U.S. Cities. Int J Environ Res Public Health 2021;18(9):4801.
57. Michelozzi P, de' Donato FK, Bargagli AM, et al. Surveillance of Summer Mortality and Preparedness to Reduce the Health Impact of Heat Waves in Italy. Int J Environ Res Public Health 2010;7(5):2256–73.
58. Giles LV, Barn P, Künzli N, et al. From Good Intentions to Proven Interventions: Effectiveness of Actions to Reduce the Health Impacts of Air Pollution. Environ Health Perspect 2011;119(1):29–36.
59. Aksa FI, Afrian R. Community adaptation strategies toward tidal flood: A Case study in Langsa, Indonesia. Jàmbá J Disaster Risk Stud 2022;14(1):1258.
60. Radhakrishnan M, Nguyen HQ, Gersonius B, et al. Coping capacities for improving adaptation pathways for flood protection in Can Tho. Vietnam. Clim Change 2018;149(1):29–41.

Moving?

Make sure your subscription moves with you!

To notify us of your new address, find your **Clinics Account Number** (located on your mailing label above your name), and contact customer service at:

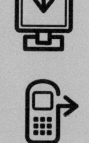

Email: journalscustomerservice-usa@elsevier.com

800-654-2452 (subscribers in the U.S. & Canada)
314-447-8871 (subscribers outside of the U.S. & Canada)

Fax number: 314-447-8029

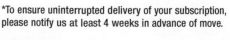

Elsevier Health Sciences Division
Subscription Customer Service
3251 Riverport Lane
Maryland Heights, MO 63043

*To ensure uninterrupted delivery of your subscription, please notify us at least 4 weeks in advance of move.

Printed and bound by CPI Group (UK) Ltd, Croydon, CR0 4YY

03/10/2024

01040469-0011